BEAUTY40+

24 BEAUTIFUL STEP-BY-STEP LOOKS

BORIS ENTRUP

BEAUTY40+
24 BEAUTIFUL STEP-BY-STEP LOOKS

PHOTOS BY
DENISE KRENTZ & ULF KRENTZ

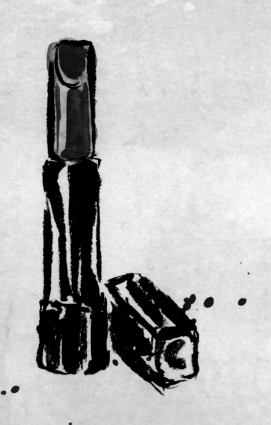

Contents

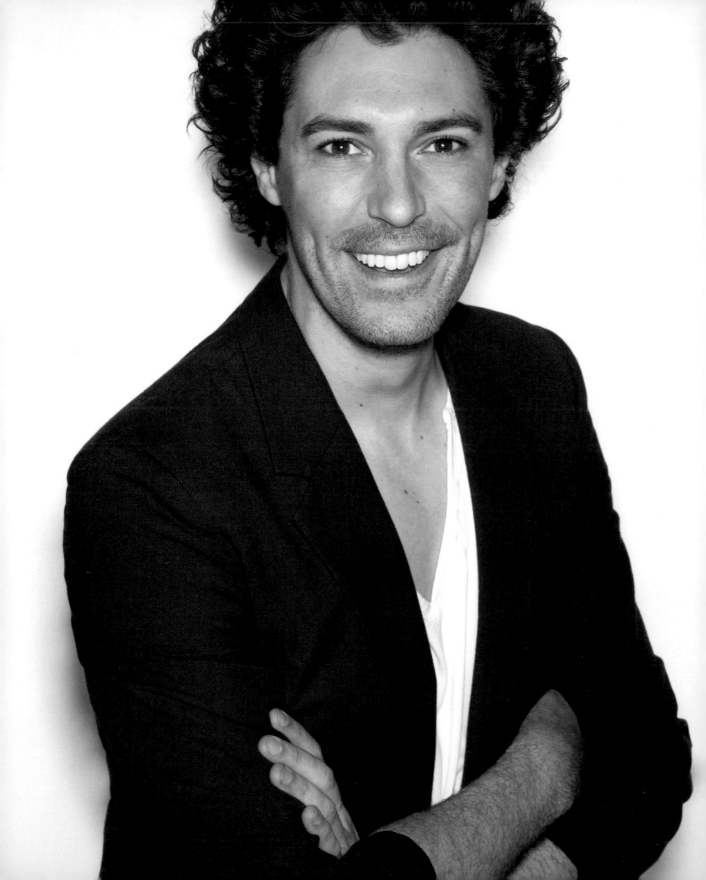

Beauty is not a question of age

Beauty is subjective. And that is why every woman is beautiful in her own way, whatever her style or age. The important thing is for women to feel good about their appearance and their individual style. And there's no need to leave it to chance when make-up gives you so many wonderful options. Make-up is my passion, because I never cease to be fascinated by the sensational effects that can be created in minutes, using simple products and tools.

Of course, this applies equally to women aged over 40, 50, or 60 years. The ultimate aim is not to look as young as possible, but simply to look as good as possible. Your skin has different needs at every age, and there are plenty of tips and tricks for staying beautiful in every phase of life. Nor should being a certain age require you to be more restrained or inconspicuous. Quite the contrary – as you go through life, you get to know yourself better; you find out what suits you, what brings out your best features, and you know what you like.

Audrey Hepburn eloquently hit the nail on the head, saying: "A woman's true beauty increases with age." My recommendation is to abandon your preconceptions about age, make-up, and styling. Make-up is fun, and it always will be.

In this book I have assembled looks for all kinds of occasions, along with ideas and tips to help you feel self-confident, assured, and beautiful. There are secret make-up tips to conceal droopy eyelids, make fine wrinkles less noticeable, or to bring radiance back to a tired complexion; cleansing routines that guarantee soft and smooth skin; nutritional tips to help the body glow from within; and hair care tricks to add greater volume, shine, and suppleness. All of this will be demonstrated using thirteen wonderful women. Four of them tell you more about themselves in their own personal portraits, relating their beauty secrets and revealing what keeps them young.

Let yourself be inspired by me and by the women in this book: be a bit daring, make a change to your make-up routine, feel free to experiment – and discover your own everyday beauty completely afresh.

Have fun!
Yours

Boris Entrup

Our models

Beauty and radiance have no age limits, as shown by our thirteen models. With their commitment and stories, each one of them has contributed to this book being an homage to the 40+ woman.

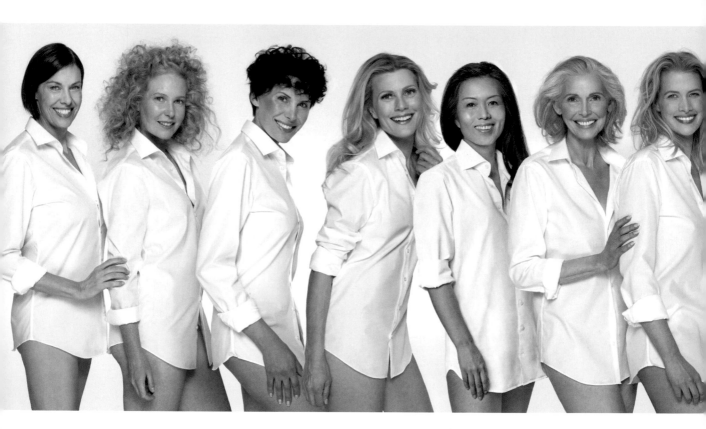

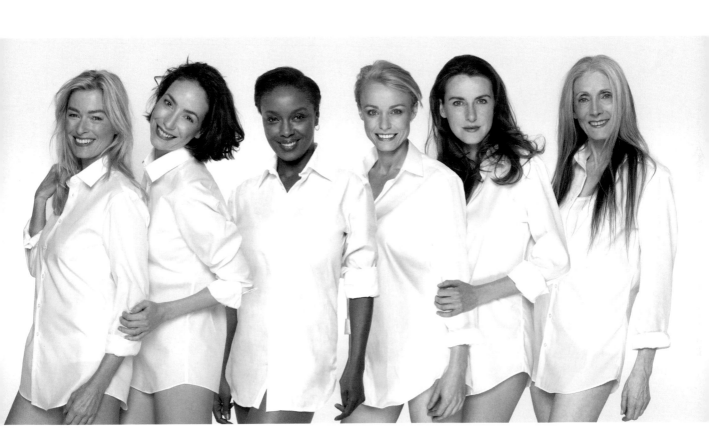

Almuth, Marion, Marzena, Ingrid, Anna, Barbara, Kerry, Martina, Esther, Caprice, Julia, Carolina, Eveline

Top 20 rejuvenators

We cannot stop time or turn back the clock. But there are any number of little tricks in the realms of make-up and styling that can make women appear younger and more radiant. I'll reveal the best ones right at the very start.

1 A natural blush

Many women are nervous about too much colour or rosy cheeks, so they opt for blusher in terracotta or apricot shades. But blusher that has a delicate pink or rosewood pigment, and therefore a translucent appearance, looks far more natural. Why? Gently pinch your cheek. The resulting shade is fresh and just as nature intended. And this is exactly what the pink and pale rose hues imitate.

2 New radiance

If you're feeling tired and your whole face shows it use a matte lipstick in a blue-toned red colour. This suits every woman, from blondes to brunettes; it doesn't needlessly make narrow lips look even smaller; and it has the optical effect of making your teeth look whiter.

3 A fringe makes you look younger

Worry lines on your forehead? Crow's feet around your eyes? The answer doesn't have to be filler and Botox – your hairdresser can help instead. A fringe is a great solution for concealing these in a way that is elegant and stylish. Note: the fringe should not be too short, but cut at an angle and falling to one side, to avoid looking too severe.

4 Arched eyebrows

Don't shape your eyebrows to be too straight. A slight curve, extending upwards for two-thirds of the length and then gently sloping down again, helps open up the eyes. It also makes droopy eyelids less noticeable (more on this on p.44).

5 No more matte

Matte, powdery foundation is best suited to young women with oily and combination skin. Unfortunately, on more mature women it can easily make the complexion appear pale and lifeless, because it emphasizes wrinkles and makes the skin look older. The same applies to heavy matte powders. It is better to use a foundation with a gentle glow and translucent powder with subtle mineralized shimmery pigments (but not glitter).

6 Beautiful camouflage

Concealer is a make-up bag essential, because it is so versatile. It covers shadows under the eyes, conceals fine lines around the mouth and nose, can make your nose look smaller and, quite simply, its luminosity gives you a more youthful complexion (more on this on p.17).

7 Bare not brown

Foundation has the task of evening out your complexion and concealing tiny flaws, but on no account should it make you appear tanned. To avoid this, you should never use a foundation that is too dark. It won't make you look more beautiful or any younger, and it can often be detected in the transition to the lighter skin on the neck. The correct shades correspond to those of your natural skin tone, or even a shade lighter (more on this on p.16). Take care when shopping: some foundations oxidize over the course of the day, becoming darker in appearance.

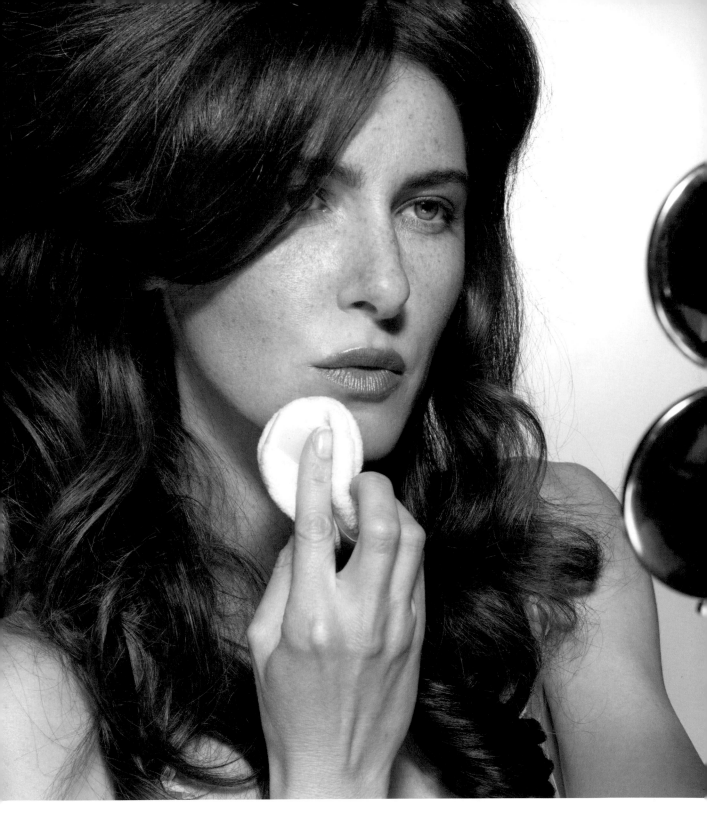

8 Try a different lip liner

Instead of using lip liner in the same shade as your lipstick, try a pencil that matches your own lip colour. This will make your lips appear larger and more even, and you can balance out the shape very slightly without it being noticeable. A touch of gloss will enhance this effect even further.

9 In the blink of an eye

Patches or tapes can help in the case of droopy eyelids. These wafer-thin, invisible, disposable adhesive strips are stuck in the eyelid crease. They pull the skin slightly upwards so that the upper section of the eyelid no longer overlaps the lower section, and the upper eyelash line is once again completely visible. Several manufacturers produce them and a pack of 64 costs around £20.

10 A riot of colour

Hollywood leads the way here. Instead of dressing in black, celebrities over the age of 40 are these days opting specifically for colour. A dress in a rich ruby shade or a vibrant emerald green delivers instant, unmissable impact on the red carpet. Luminescent yellow has a similarly sensational effect.

11 Soft lines

Very sharply drawn eyeliner can look severe, which makes you appear older. A far better way of accentuating the upper and lower lash lines is to use a softer kohl or kajal pencil, or alternatively a powder eyeshadow. Both of these can be blended using a foam applicator or blender brush, for a much softer look that makes you appear younger as a result (more on this on p.37).

12 Natural nails

Nails in nude shades or with a French manicure make your hands appear longer, and cleverly draw attention away from the little lines and spots of pigmentation on the backs of your hands.

13 Luscious lips

So-called lip plumpers (a special type of lip gloss) are a great option for temporarily achieving fuller lips. As well as containing nourishing substances, lip plumpers include ingredients such as chilli, menthol, or cinnamon, which stimulate increased circulation in the lips. This results in a deeper colour, a more distinct outline, and a plumper appearance. Depending on the quantity of active circulation-stimulating substances in the lip plumper, the lips may prickle for a short time, or even burn slightly. The effect lasts for around 2 to 4 hours. Coloured lip plumpers are also available, so you can do without lipstick.

14 Bronzer brings sunshine to your face

… if you use it to shade the temples, cheekbones, and lower parts of the cheeks in a C-shape. Never apply too much to the centre of your face, as this can look unnatural, which will make you look older.

15 The feathered look

Watch out: once you're in your mid-40s, your hairdresser may recommend "something practical" and try to persuade you into a "smart" shorter haircut. But a so-called shag cut is a softer and younger look than most short styles. It's a feathered, layered cut, which falls somewhere between chin and shoulder length, gently framing the face. Bobs and other geometric cuts are less flattering by contrast, as they further accentuate the increasingly angular facial structure.

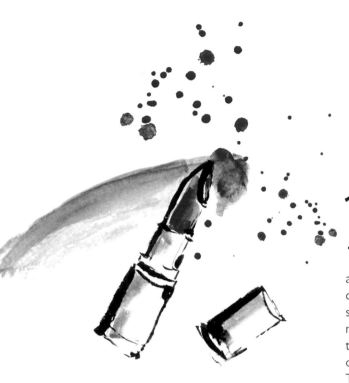

18 Create contours

The skin on your face (and indeed the rest of your body) gradually loses its subcutaneous fat tissues. This substance functions as a kind of internal padding and has the effect of smoothing out your skin. As it diminishes, the face can appear more haggard, and the skin is no longer so youthful and firm. Make a virtue of necessity and accentuate your facial contours beneath the cheekbones. Blusher applied to the highest part of the cheekbone further emphasizes the facial structure. The overall effect works beautifully: cheekbones are accentuated and facial contours are enhanced.

16 Not too tight-lipped

Over time, our lips become thinner because the skin is drier and the padding provided by subcutaneous fat tissue diminishes. Lipsticks in dark red or brown shades just compound this impression. Better options are brighter berry colours that reflect the natural lip colour and are, at most, a couple of shades darker.

17 Moisture is everything

Particularly with dry skin, your complexion can appear matte and dull as the day progresses. Rub a little bit of day cream between your palms and press the flat of your hands gently over your whole face; your skin will instantly absorb the moisture and be radiant again. This works wonderfully over make-up too.

19 Off-tones for the eyelids

Women with lines around their eyes are often cautious about using shimmery eye shadow colours – but this caution is completely unfounded. Colours with a gentle shimmer bring more light to the face than matte shades. The colour is crucial: greys and browns, and natural-looking off-tones such as taupe, stone, or mauve are particularly flattering.

20 Eighty per cent is enough

Don't be too perfect with your make-up and styling. Anything that is applied too precisely may have an ageing effect. Aim for the more spontaneous approach preferred by younger women: your ponytail can happily look a bit messy, and some casually dabbed-on coloured lip gloss often looks fresher than precisely outlined lips.

Make-up
Looks
and Basics

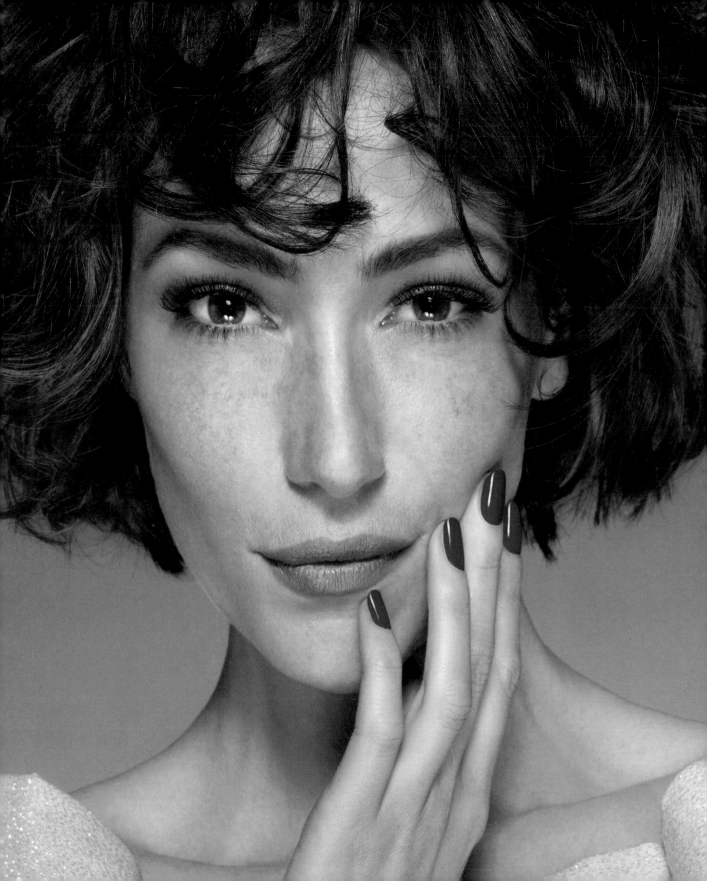

FOUNDATION & CONCEALER

These two complexion flatterers form the basis of every look and also discreetly conceal small blemishes – lines, circles under the eyes, red blotches, and so on. This section reveals how to use them and how to select the appropriate shade.

FOUNDATION

Foundation prepares your face for subsequent make-up steps. Anti-ageing foundations, with their light-reflecting pigments and nourishing ingredients, are ideal for more mature skin, or alternatively you can use BB (blemish balm) or CC (colour correcting) creams, which are a cross between a foundation and a tinted moisturizer.

The important thing to remember when choosing the colour is that excessively dark shades have an ageing effect; the colour should match your natural skin tone. Always test make-up on an unmade-up cheek, not on the back of your hand. If the colour blends in with your own skin tone, then you have found the correct shade.

SOFT FOCUS

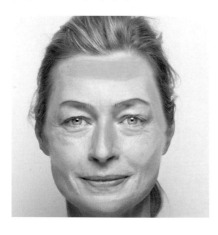 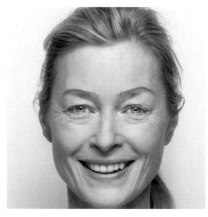

1 Preparation: Allow your daily moisturizing cream to absorb, then apply foundation and carefully work into the skin using fingers, a small make-up sponge, or a brush.

2 Blending: Take care that no colour is caught between the eyebrows and that there are no edges at the hairline, ears, or where the chin meets the neck.

CONCEALER

If there is one make-up product that a woman over 40 cannot do without, it is concealer. This exceptionally versatile product provides perfect cover for any under-eye shadows; it virtually magics away lines, wrinkles, and irregularities; it enhances skin tone; and works as a highlighter, so that your complexion and eyes can really shine. Importantly, there are different concealers for different purposes. Products with antibacterial ingredients are ideal for concealing blemishes and simultaneously speeding up the healing process. However, these may have a drying effect on the delicate eye area, where liquid or cream concealers with nourishing ingredients are a better choice. Always use as little product as possible, as any excess will collect in the creases, making them more visible.

TIPS & TRICKS

In order for concealer to disguise skin blemishes and not draw attention to them, you need to select an appropriate shade. The colour should be one shade lighter than your natural skin tone and must match the skin's undertone, which will be either yellow, red, or olive. Spots and redness can be completely concealed using a green-coloured concealer, since green "absorbs" the complementary red colour. Bluish shadows under the eyes, on the other hand, are best disguised with a yellow- or orange-tinted shade. In all cases apply the product in an extremely thin layer and work it into the skin by dabbing rather than stroking with your finger.

RETOUCHING

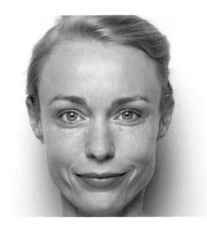

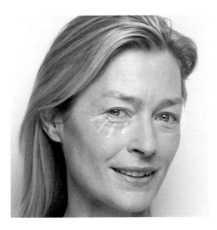

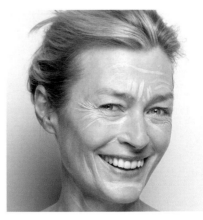

Shadows under the eyes disappear if you dab concealer onto the lower eyelid and pat it in. Tip: also apply to the inner corner of the eye – this makes the eyes seem more alert.

Any puffiness beneath the eyes will be less conspicuous if concealer is applied in radial lines from the lower lid down to the cheekbone and then blended into the skin.

More pronounced wrinkles can be made to appear less deep by using a lighter concealer. Apply the concealer selectively – too much product will just draw more attention to the wrinkles.

GOLDEN SHADOW

Warm shades, such as bronze, gold, and copper, are wonderful for creating a harmonious and natural make-up style. As an added bonus, they conjure up a fresh, sun-kissed complexion.

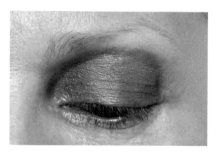

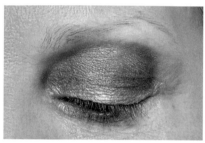

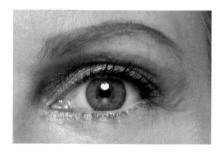

1 LIDS

Cover the entire eyelid, to just above the crease, with a copper-coloured, shimmery eyeshadow.

2 LASH LINE

Draw a wide line along the upper lash line using a gold-coloured eyeshadow. This visually opens up the eyes if the lids are droopy, and helps emphasize the lashes.

3 EYEBROWS

Apply mascara. Use an eyebrow brush to trace the eyebrows with a pale brown eyebrow powder, and shape them.

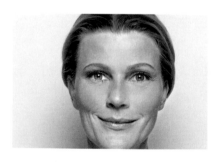

4 CHEEKS

Use a blusher brush to apply and then blend in a bronze-coloured blusher (or a bronzer) over the cheekbones towards the nasolabial fold.

RED CHEEKS?

If you want to use blusher but you have problems with skin redness, perhaps due to rosacea, there is a fundamental rule to follow: before applying blusher, make sure that you even out your complexion in the affected area with a concealer, a strongly pigmented foundation, or a mineral foundation (which can be applied in multiple layers without appearing mask-like on the skin).

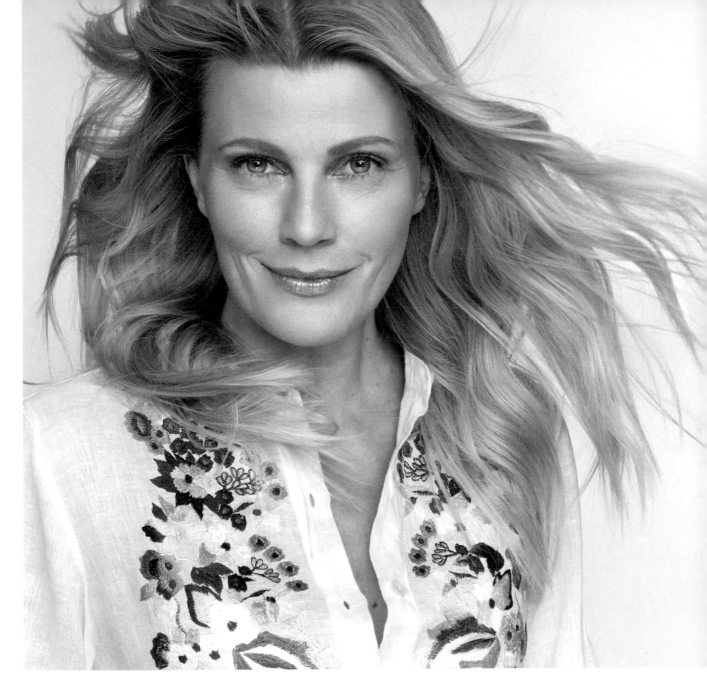

The highest point for eyeshadow should always be located immediately above the pupils; this makes your eyes look clearer and more alert.

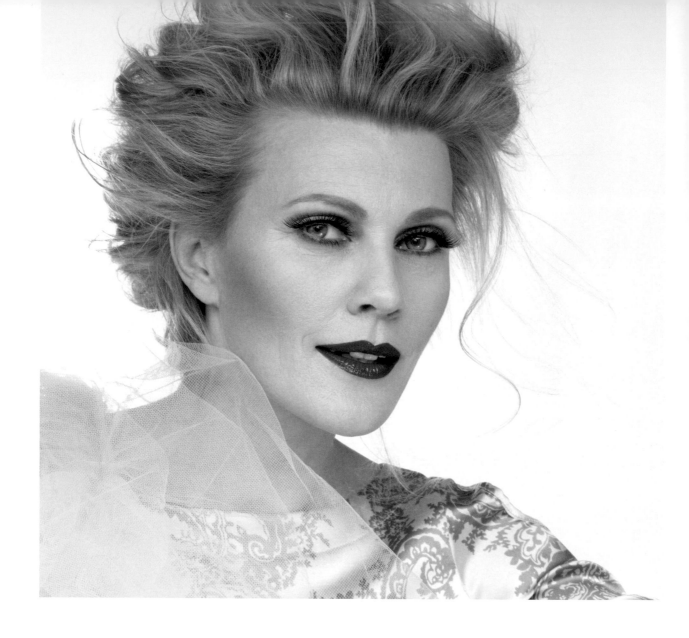

FIRST LADY

Expressive, smoky eyes are a real attention grabber. Here they contribute to a fabulous and extremely flattering evening look for Ingrid, providing a perfect contrast to her delicate complexion and pastel silk outfit.

For very thin lips, a lighter berry shade is a better choice than a darker blackberry colour, which makes the mouth look smaller.

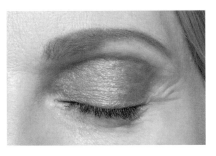

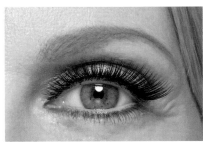

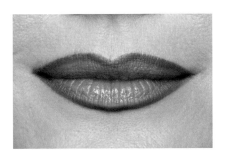

1 EYELIDS

Use an eye-shadow brush to apply a glossy grey-mauve eyeshadow over the whole eyelid, and blend it out slightly over the crease.

2 EYELASHES

Emphasize the eyelid crease and lower lash line with an anthracite-coloured eyeshadow. An even more dramatic look can be created by adding false eyelashes.

3 CONTOURS

Use a lip pencil to outline first the upper lip and then the lower in a colour similar to your lipstick. It's better to go a shade lighter rather than darker.

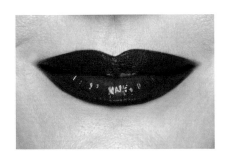

4 LIPS

Apply an intense red lipstick. This is best done with a lip brush. Finally, dab a little gloss onto the centre of the lips.

THE LOOK

False eyelashes open up your eyes. If you like the effect, a semi-permanent eyelash extension or thickening procedure done by a professional might be worth investigating. The process involves inserting between 80 and 200 individual lashes among your own eyelashes, and does away with the need for mascara. This glorious effect lasts for around 4 weeks before the whole thing needs to be replaced.

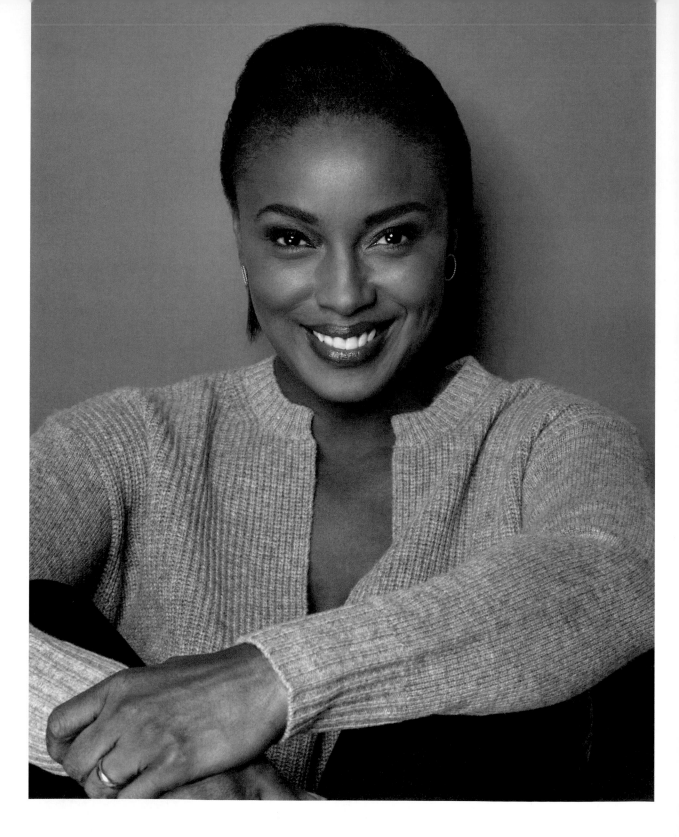

SHINY NUDES

In the right tones nude shades can look gorgeous and make the skin glow, even if you have a dark complexion. Use shimmering tones in combination with subtle highlights to create shape and definition.

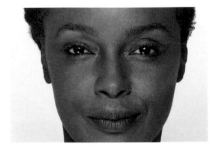

1 PRIMER

Apply liquid foundation. Use a highlighting concealer on the nose, under the eyes and eyebrows, on the centre of the top lip, and at the highest point of the cheekbones.

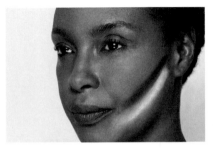

2 CONTOUR

Apply a dark contouring powder below the highest point of the cheekbones, then apply a highlight under it, along the jaw line. Blend using a brush.

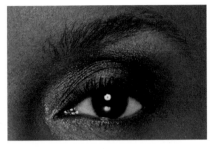

3 EYES

Apply a taupe eyeshadow across the whole eyelid, then apply a darker tone of shadow in the crease. Put mascara on the upper lashes only.

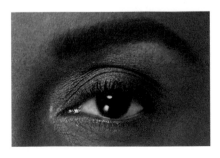

4 EYEBROWS

Fill eyebrows with brow powder and smooth with brow gel. Draw a soft line with brown eyeliner on the upper lash line. Highlight above the pupil with a gold eyeshadow.

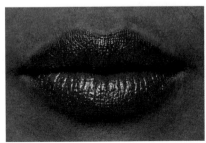

5 LIPS

Outline the lips using a dark lipliner to suit. The ratio of lower to upper lip should be about the same. Dab on a little lip gloss.

CONTOURING

So-called shaping or contouring is a fantastic trick that lets you play with light and shadows. Darker areas blend into the background or make for sharper outlines, while lighter areas add emphasis and create a three-dimensional effect.

TOOLKIT

You need two products for contouring: a skin-coloured foundation for the base layer and make-up that is one or two shades darker for shading. Beginners should start with a light liquid foundation and a darker foundation stick, a combination that works particularly well. Specialized contouring products are also available in stick, cream, or powder form.

STEP 1: HIGHLIGHTS

Add highlights using the lighter shade under the eyes, between the eyebrows, on the forehead, on the ridge of the nose, and on the chin. Blend the make-up well with your fingers, a small make-up sponge, or a large foundation brush, so that it blends perfectly with your skin tone.

STEP 2: DARKER SHADING

Now use the darker shade for sculpting. It should be applied to the temples and under the cheekbones to make the face appear narrower and to emphasize the bone structure. When applied to the forehead, it makes it appear shorter, and when dabbed on the sides of the nostrils, the nose looks narrower. Any ill-defined contours in the area between chin and neck can be concealed in the same way.

STEP 3: FINISHING

Now blend in the darker shaded areas by gently stroking the blobs and strips of make-up and working them into the skin. Finally, apply a mid-toned shade of powder to the areas between the highlights and the darker shading.

TIPS & TRICKS

Be especially careful to thoroughly blend the transitional areas between the highlights and darker shading – otherwise your make-up trickery will be detected immediately. It also helps if the make-up products you use are not too shiny or red-toned in colour. Cool, neutral browns are perfect. Always check the final effect in daylight and never only under artificial light.

MODELLING FACIAL STRUCTURE

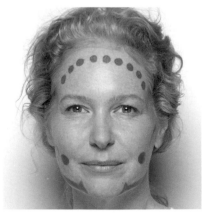

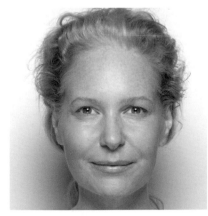

Angular face: Curved blobs of darker shading shorten Marion's high forehead. Dark foundation along the edges of the chin and at the extended corners of the mouth help give a softer appearance to her face.

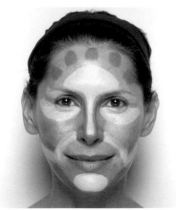

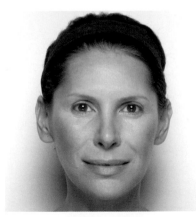

Heart-shaped face: Highlights on the forehead, nose, chin, and beneath the eyes bring radiance to Marzena's face and make her nose look slimmer. Darker shading on the forehead makes her face appear more oval in shape.

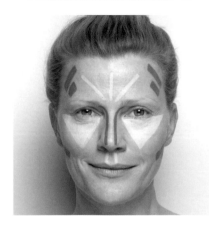

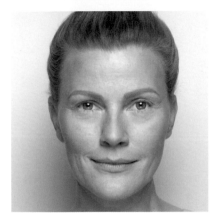

Oval face: Highlights beneath the eyes ensure that Ingrid looks vibrant and any small wrinkles are less noticeable. Darker shading at the temples helps balance her facial proportions, and shading beneath the cheekbones emphasizes them.

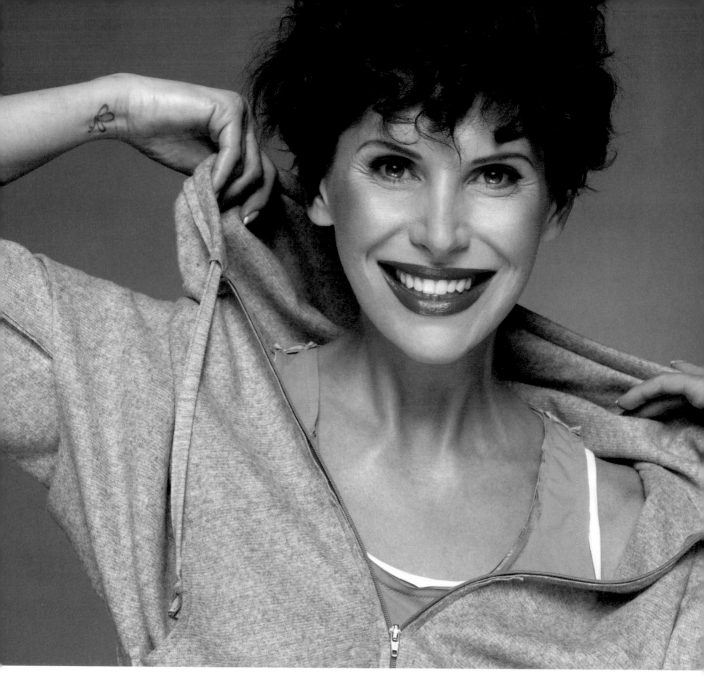

When applying strong lipstick colours, you need to be careful to work precisely. Blurred edges look inelegant and may make you seem older.

FRESH & EASY

Bright lip colours are like a wake-up call for your whole face. Have the courage to try a luscious mandarin orange some time. It suits brunettes and blondes alike and is especially flattering for narrow lips.

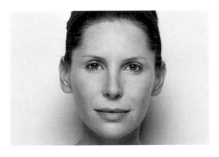

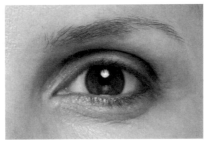

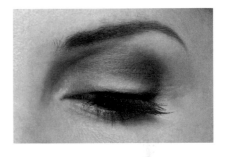

1 HIGHLIGHTS
After applying a base foundation, add highlights (using concealer or a paler foundation) to the chin, central forehead, under the eyes, and the bridge of the nose. This creates a 3-D effect.

2 EYELIDS
Apply a flesh-toned eyeshadow over the entire eyelid. This will really show off the eyelashes once mascara is applied.

3 EYEBROWS
Blend a golden-brown eyeshadow from the outer corner of the eye up into the crease. Draw a thin line along the lid and apply plenty of mascara. Delicately fill in the eyebrows using an eyebrow pencil.

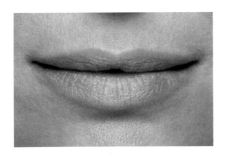

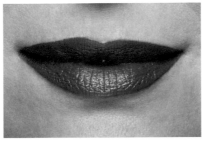

4 PREPARATION
To make your lipstick last longer, apply a lip primer to the lips and trace the outline using a clear lip liner.

5 LIPS
Carefully apply mandarin-coloured lipstick using a lip brush. Dab a bit of clear gloss onto the centre of the lips to make them look fresher.

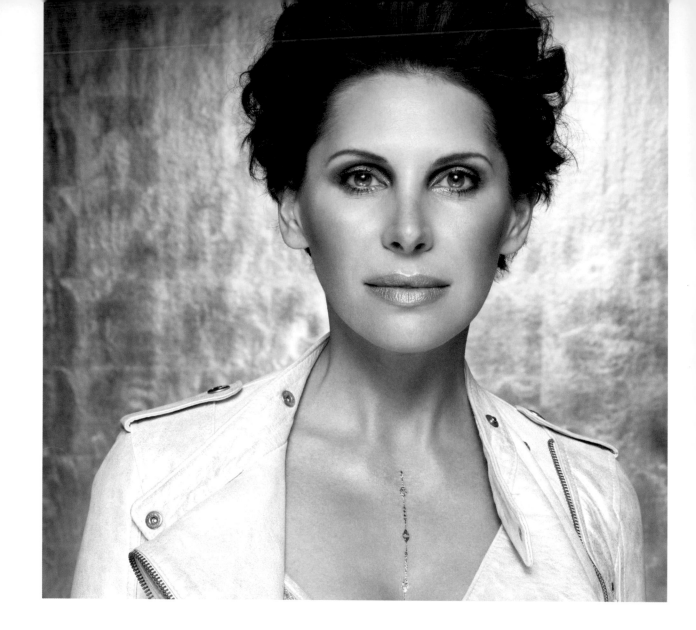

EMPOWERED WOMEN

Marzena's gamine style gets a hint of femininity and a dash of rock 'n' roll with this strong but not overly colourful look.

If you naturally have more strongly pigmented skin, shadows under the eyes can be particularly noticeable. A not too bright, yellow- or olive-toned concealer is a quick remedy.

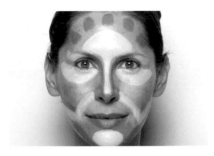

1 CONTOURING

Darker shading gives shape to the face and blends into the background. Highlights add emphasis and even out any redness or shadows. This enhances the facial structure.

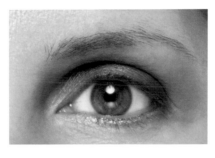

2 FOUNDATION

To make the eyeshadow last longer, apply a base layer of eye primer over the entire eyelid. Then apply a cool, grey-violet shadow up into the eyelid crease.

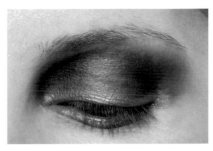

3 SHADING

Emphasize the crease using a grey-brown eyeshadow, softening the central lid area with a brush. Then trace the lash line in gold and add highlights above the pupil.

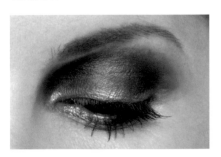

4 EMPHASIS

Apply mascara generously to the eyelashes, focusing on the base of the lashes. Fill out the eyebrows using a medium-brown eyebrow powder, and coax into shape with an eyebrow brush.

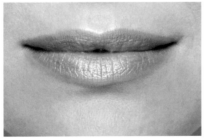

5 ADD VOLUME

Nude-coloured lipsticks and a dab of gloss in the centre of the lips create the illusion of greater volume. Emphasize the cupid's bow of the upper lip with a beige kohl liner.

BLUSHER & BRONZER

Blusher and bronzer give your skin a freshness boost, create a healthy-looking, radiant complexion, or a sun-kissed skin tone. What's more, you can use them to create a more sculpted and well-proportioned facial structure.

THE CORRECT SHADE

Rule of thumb: the most natural blush effect is created using delicate pink and rose hues. But other shades can also look fantastic. Apricot, for instance, gives a fresh and healthy look; cool bluish tones come across as very sophisticated; and terracotta shades will give you the "I've just been on holiday" look.

THE RIGHT CONSISTENCY

Blusher is available as a powder, in cream form, as a mousse, or as a liquid. Powder blush is particularly easy to apply with a brush and lasts for a long time. Cream and mousse blushers are applied with fingers or a brush. Liquid blusher is rather trickier to apply, as it dries very quickly on the skin.

THE PERFECT TECHNIQUE

Take some mousse blusher with your fingers and blend it over the cheeks using small circular movements. Liquid blusher should be dabbed on and blended in quickly.

For powder blusher, collect some product on the blusher brush by moving it in a circular fashion so that the powder particles also find their way inside the brush. To remove any excess powder, gently tap the brush on the side of your hand, test in the palm of your hand how much colour the brush will deliver. Then apply to the cheeks, check the result in the mirror, and if necessary apply a further one or two layers.

TIPS & TRICKS

Too much blusher? Cream or mousse can be softened by blending them in a bit more. For powder blusher, add a dab of liquid or compact foundation to dilute the colour. A general purpose blender brush (see pp.152–153) may also help: use small circular movements from the outside inwards to soften the colour.

APPLYING BLUSHER ACCURATELY

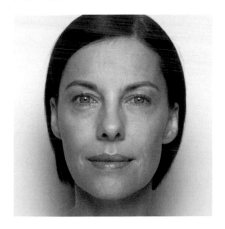

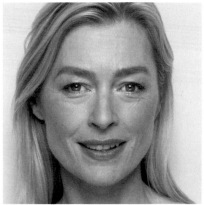

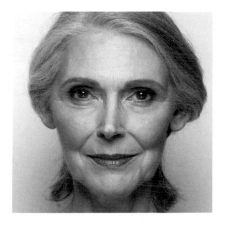

To add structure: Apply blusher beneath the highest point of the cheekbone and then blend towards the hairline to the temples and to the corners of the mouth.

For a really fresh look: Apply the blusher (preferably pink, peach, or coral) directly to the highest point of the cheekbone.

To help distract from wrinkles: A delicate peach tone applied to the cheekbones draws attention to the eyes and nose, and away from the mouth area.

APPLYING BRONZER CORRECTLY

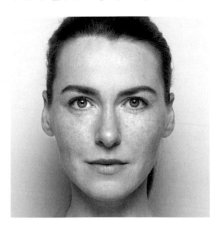

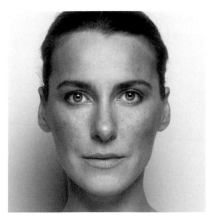

Before: Carolina has a wonderfully delicate complexion, but sometimes looks a little pale.

After: Apply bronzing powder to those areas that would be tanned by the sun.

"Live for today!"

Life has something to offer every single day; it is full of little moments of joy – sometimes it takes a major crisis to make you appreciate this …

Anyone who sees Marzena, relaxed and without make-up in her T-shirt and jeans, might well imagine she was in her early to mid-30s. Her short dark hair, attentive eyes, and warm smile make the now 43-year-old appear much younger. But 19 years ago she wasn't counting on necessarily even celebrating her 40th birthday. It all started with a series of frequent infections. Marzena felt listless and lacking in energy, permanently tired and increasingly weak, until one day she collapsed at a family celebration. But doctors could not work out what was wrong. Marzena cut back her working hours in an attempt to recover and to find enough energy for her then 4-year-old daughter Vivien. When her condition still failed to improve over a prolonged period, the doctors repeated their investigations. The diagnosis was a shock: cancer of the lymph nodes.

"When the doctor asked me about my family, I realized this was something really serious …"

Marzena remembers that, shortly before the diagnosis, she had driven past a huge billboard for a fashion company she had modelled for. "The situation was completely ridiculous: first this glamorous photograph – and then ten minutes later I was sitting opposite the doctor, being asked if I had any family. That's when I realized this was something really serious." After the diagnosis Marzena was completely numb, running past her husband, out of the surgery and onto the

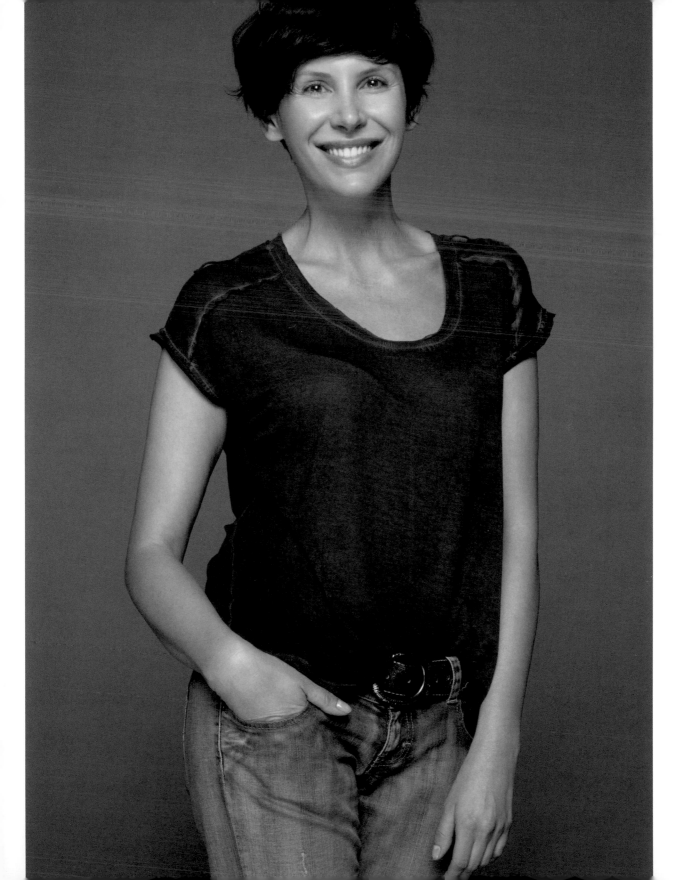

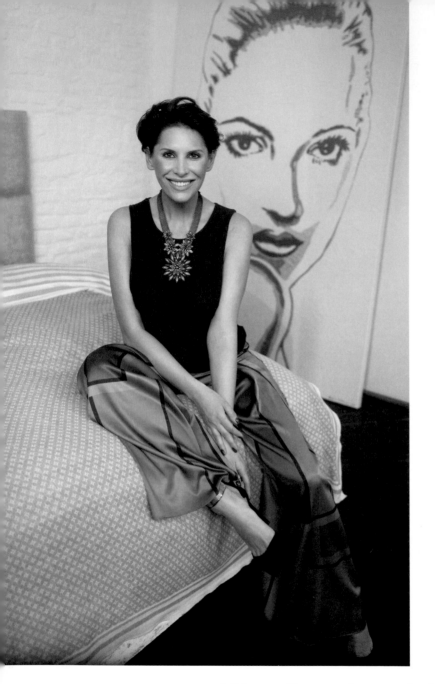

street. She was not even able to cry. She says, "It was like I'd been turned to stone. I just kept thinking of my little daughter, who was possibly going to have to grow up without a mother."

The doctors proposed a combined therapy of radiation and high-dose chemotherapy. This poisonous cocktail, aimed at conquering the cancer, sapped her of all her energy and caused extreme nausea and hair loss. "In the first few days after chemo it took a huge effort just to move the bedcovers to one side. I couldn't even begin to contemplate standing up," she remembers. Marzena was lucky: she responded well to the treatment and the tumour shrank visibly.

"I enjoy today with all my senses"

Today Marzena is considered to be cured. But she knows that with cancer you can never be quite sure: "Sometimes cancer cells lie dormant in your body for years or decades, only to strike again." Above all, Marzena has learned one thing from her illness: life is happening now. And you can't predict the future. "Even when I got my cancer diagnosis, the first thing I did was pull out my planner to check when I would be through with chemo and able to work again." Since then, she's learned to just let things happen as they will. "The illness has forced me, albeit in a rather drastic manner, to sometimes chill out a bit more." Today she lives her life with greater candour and attentiveness, and she knows when she needs time out or more space for herself. She also pays more attention to her diet. "Previously I would often have just stuffed some food inside me, without giving it a second thought. Today I really appreciate mealtimes and now and again I try to eat an apple in between, properly taking time to enjoy it. I sniff it, calmly cut it up, and then savour it with all my senses. Of course I don't always manage this, but I do increasingly succeed," she laughs. "I now know life is simply too good not to be enjoyed every single day."

EXERCISE

Creating more space for yourself

In the hurly-burly of everyday life it is not always possible to be mindful and to create the freedom and space you really need. The following exercise can help you create a feeling of greater space for yourself. Use it at times when you quite literally feel constricted, or in situations that are psychologically challenging due to stress, grief, or anger.

Stand up tall with legs hip-width apart. The soles of your feet should be planted firmly and securely on the floor; knees can be slightly bent. Now bend both arms slightly, the right arm should hover at around stomach height a few centimetres away from your body, the left arm should be roughly at chest height. The aim is to look as though you are giving yourself a hug at a slight distance. Now alternate the arms so that the right arm is at chest height, the left hovering in front of your belly button; this time make the distance from your body slightly greater. Repeat the exercise, continuing to alternate arms, and gradually increasing the distance between arms and body until you have a gap that feels good, and you can imagine your body expanding to give yourself a greater sense of space and awareness.

EYESHADOW & EYELINER

Two truly magical products for creating a more youthful appearance. They can instantly make small eyes seem larger, eradicate any traces of fatigue, conceal droopy eyelids, and distract from fine wrinkles.

EYESHADOWS

Applying make-up so your eyes seem larger is really easy: use a pale eyeshadow to cover the entire eyelid and then add some darker shading to the eyelid crease. Some highlights beneath the eyebrows and kohl pencil at the corners of the eyes immediately create a more open expression.

If the eyelids are droopy, it is important to make sure the eyeshadow can be seen when the eyes are open, in order to achieve an optical lifting effect. To do this, apply the eyeshadow beyond the eyelid crease. Dark colours are more effective here than lighter shades.

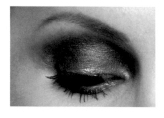
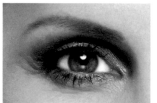

Intense: Violet eye shadow over the eyelid and on the lower lash line makes the eyes look larger. Gold highlights at the inner corner of the eye, along the lash line, and in the centre of the eyelid will open up the eyes still further.

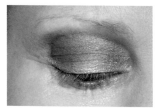
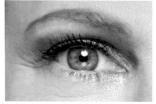

Radiant: Warm hues on the eyelid, in combination with gold on the upper lash line, ensure a radiant look.

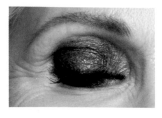
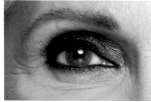

Smoky: To add definition to the eyes and make them more visible, work with dark eyeshadows, but take care not to extend colour beyond the corners of the eyes.

EYELINER & KOHL

Many women steer clear of eyeliner, afraid they won't be able to draw a neat line, or that the effect will be too harsh. Have no fear: when it comes to applying eyeliner, help is available. And when it is drawn with a kohl liner and then softened, eyeliner has a much more muted effect. It is best to use a cream kohl that becomes powdery after application.

FROM DRAMATIC TO SOFT

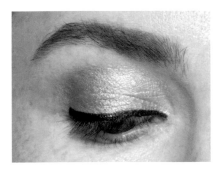

1 Draw the line: Starting at the inner corner of the eye, draw a line to the centre of the eyelid. Then draw a line to meet this from the outer corner of the eye towards the centre.

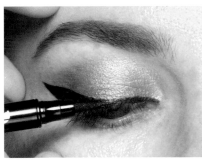

2 Draw a cat flick: Locate an end point somewhere between the outer corner of the eye and the end of your eyebrow, and join this to the line along the eyelid.

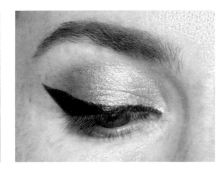

3 Filling in: Fill in the area beneath this with the eyeliner. Tip: when applying the colour, look straight ahead in the mirror and support your hand on your cheek.

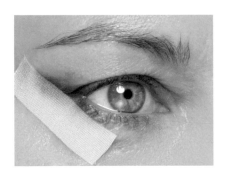

1 Fix tape in place: Stick a piece of low-tack tape from the end of the eyebrow to the outer corner of the eye, leaving a small gap to the lower lash line.

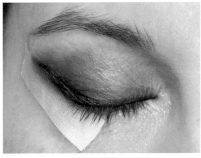

2 Position the pencil: Using kohl, draw a line right along the lash line from the inner corner of the eye. Start again from the chosen end point and connect to the line.

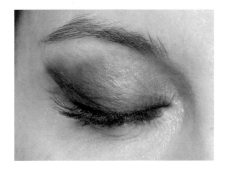

3 Soften the line: Soften the upper edge of the kohl line along the eyelid using the pencil's smudger, or a cotton bud.

SOPHISTICATED

Always emphasize your best facial features, then any tiny blemishes will be less noticeable. Carolina's strong green eyes are transformed into glimmering cat eyes using some black eyeliner and an aqua-blue kohl.

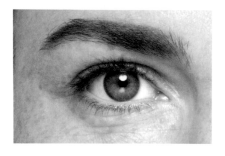

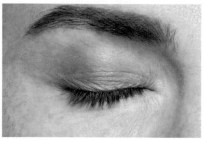

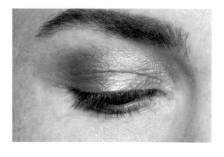

1 EYEBROWS
Fill in any gaps in the eyebrows using an eyebrow brush and some dark brown eyebrow powder, and brush into shape.

2 BASE
Apply a pale grey cream eyeshadow over the entire eyelid up to the crease. Blend in gently using your finger.

3 EYESHADOW
Before the eyeshadow is dry, apply a pearl shimmer eyeshadow powder up to the eyelid crease and blend in.

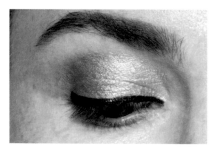

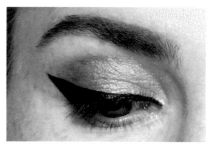

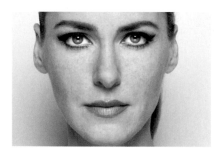

4 EYELINER 1
First position the eyeliner at the inner corner of the eye and draw a line to the centre of the lash line. Then draw a line from the outer corner of the eye to meet it in the middle.

5 EYELINER 2
Determine a spot for the end of your cat flick line, above the outer corner of the eye. Draw a line to the upper and lower lash lines and fill in the area between.

6 LIPS & LASHES
Apply an aqua-blue kohl liner along the lower lash line. Apply mascara. Outline the lips with a lip pencil and fill in with pink lipstick.

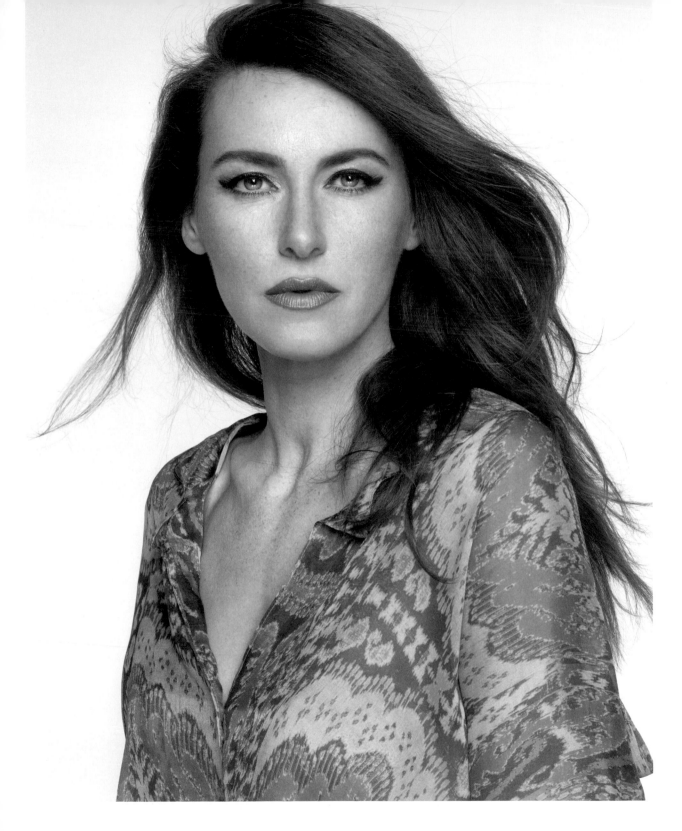

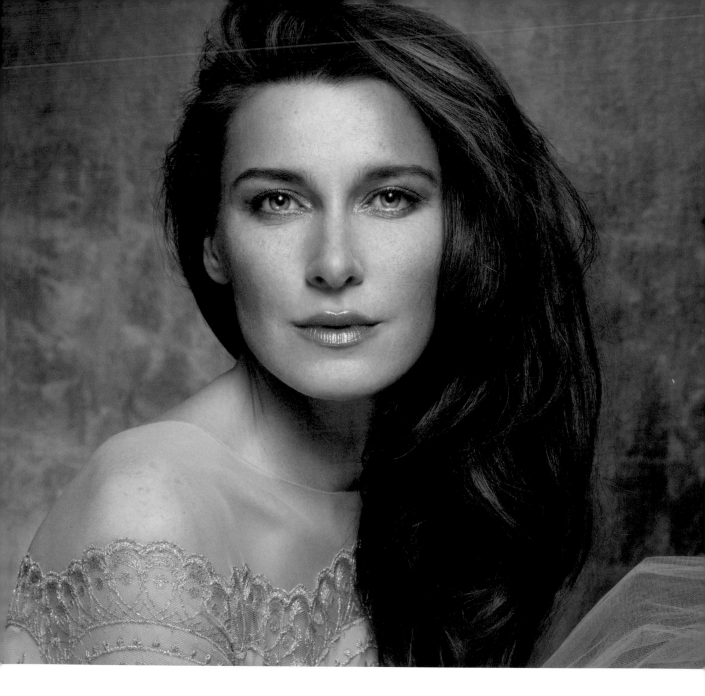

To ensure your complexion retains its beautiful lustre with this look, only apply the matte powder to the T-zone.

SUN KISSED

Naturally radiant: a clear, glowing complexion always looks more youthful than an opaque layer of make-up. Warm, shimmery metallic colours – copper, gold, and bronze – are perfect for achieving this look.

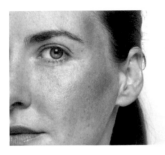 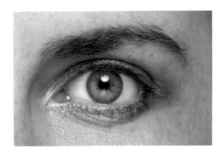 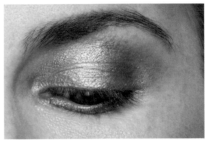

1 BRONZE

Use cream blusher in a pale pink-toned bronze shade, applying it to the cheekbones up to the temples and blending well into the skin with your fingers.

2 COPPER

Apply copper-coloured eyeshadow over the eyelid to the crease, and blend towards the outer corner of the eye using an eyeshadow brush.

3 GOLD

Apply a metallic gold eyeshadow to the centre of the eyelid above the pupil, using a small eyeshadow brush.

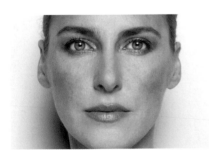

4 ROSE GOLD

Only apply mascara to the upper lashes. Apply a pinky nude lipstick and then dab on some clear lip gloss with a gold shimmer.

BRONZING ME SOFTLY

Bronzing powder is really versatile and can be used throughout the year. It is available in both loose and compact forms, and even as a brush that dispenses powder at the touch of a button. Be warned that it's vital to match the shade of bronzing powder to your own skin tone. Very strong, slightly orange shades only suit quite tanned skin; on other complexions they tend to look unnatural. For very pale skin, choose a bronzing powder that gives your complexion just a hint of colour.

MINIMALISM

Heading straight from work to an evening function? No problem. Here's a five-minute make-up routine you can achieve even in the office. For Carolina, statement lips in cherry red really brighten her complexion.

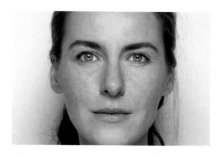

1 FOUNDATION
To freshen up your complexion, apply foundation and use concealer to disguise any shadows or discolouration, and ensure skin looks completely even.

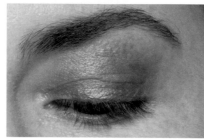

2 EYESHADOW
Apply a shimmery, taupe-coloured eyeshadow over the whole eyelid and blend in carefully with an eyeshadow brush.

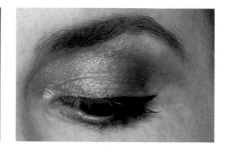

3 EYELINER
Add a highlight centrally above the pupil in a pale, shiny grey. Draw an extremely fine line with eyeliner from the centre of the eyelid to the outer corner of the eye.

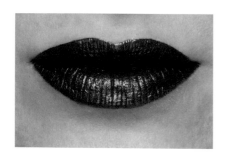

4 LIPSTICK
Outline the lips using lip liner, then fill them in with the liner to make the colour last longer. Apply cherry red lipstick using a brush.

OPPOSITES ATTRACT ...

Eyeshadows are available in countless colours. Be a bit daring and try a new one out now and again. The abiding principle is that your own eye colour is best enhanced by contrasting eyeshadows. Cool, bluish shades go well with warmer eye colours, while cooler eye colours are best complemented by warmer shades. For a powerful impact you need strong colours. Softer colours give a more muted effect.

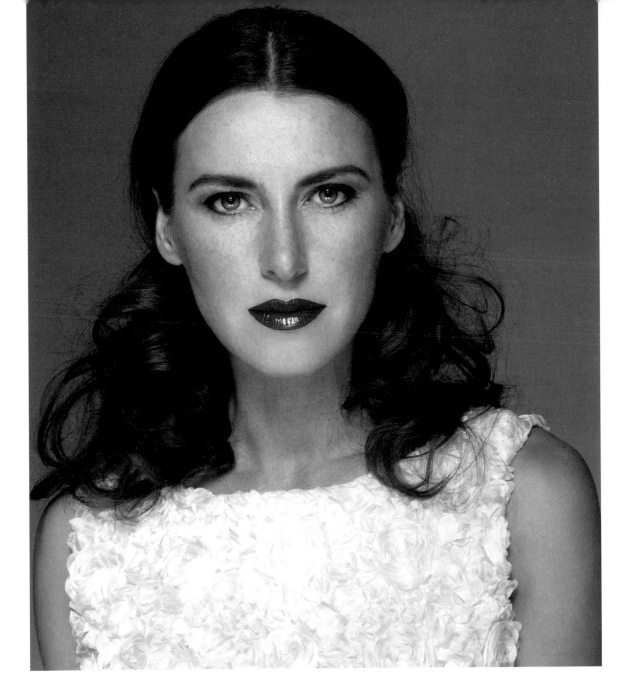

A long-lasting lipstick formula ensures that your lip colour will survive the entire evening, without having to be constantly reapplied.

EYEBROWS

Well-shaped eyebrows provide a frame for your face and can even help balance out your facial structure. Whether narrow or wide, highly arched, or straight – it is all just a matter of taste.

THE PERFECT SHAPE

Imagine a line from the outer edge of your nostril up to the inner corner of the eye. Extend this line to find the point where your eyebrow should begin. Place a pencil or an eyebrow brush in this position. Now slide it towards the pupil, with the other end still in position at the nostril. The point where it intersects with the eyebrow indicates where the highest point should be. The end of the eyebrow should coincide with an imaginary line drawn from the nostril to the outer corner of the eye.

If you pluck your eyebrows yourself, do it one hair at a time in a magnifying mirror. Every now and then, check the shape and symmetry by looking in a standard mirror. Bevelled high-quality tweezers are worth their weight in gold: they will securely grip even the finest, shortest hairs.

THE RIGHT COLOUR

The fundamental rule is that eyebrows should always match the colour of your hair. If your hair is dyed a significantly darker colour than it would be naturally, you should adjust the colour of your eyebrows accordingly. For dyed blonde hair and naturally darker eyebrows, the best approach is gentle bleaching. Light or medium cool brown eyebrows, without any hint of red, suit most people. Pale anthracite eyebrows look good with ashy or grey-coloured hair.

THE PERFECT PRODUCT

Eyebrow powder is perfect for filling in little gaps in the eyebrows. Use an eyebrow pencil to trace the brows using short, feathery strokes, or to define the upper edges. Eyebrow mascara is particularly easy to apply. It is available in clear form, for smoothing the hairs down, or in a range of colours. Just brush it once over the hairs using the applicator – and you're done!

TIPS & TRICKS

The most important thing is to focus attention on the upper edge of the eyebrow. This lifts the brow and makes the eyes appear larger and more awake. By contrast, a line along the lower edge of the eyebrows visually compresses the eyes.

EYEBROW SHAPING

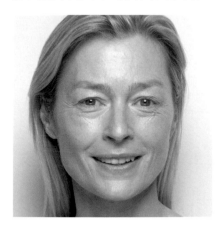

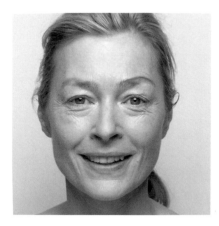

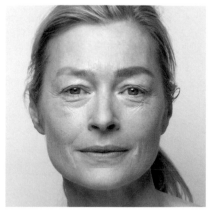

1 Preparation: Use a cotton bud or eyebrow brush to remove any possible make-up residue from the eyebrows and brush them upwards using an eyebrow brush.

2 Definition: Use a well-sharpened eyebrow pencil to neatly trace the upper brow line, bearing in mind the ideal shape (see left).

3 Filling in: Blend the line downwards using the eyebrow brush, and then fill in any small gaps with brow powder.

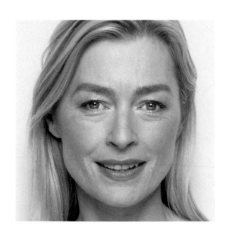

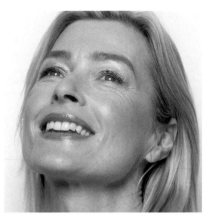

4 Balancing: Fill in the second eyebrow in the same way. Finish by shaping the eyebrows using the brush.

Perfectly shaped: Relatively wide, light brown eyebrows suit Martina wonderfully. They make her eyes really shine.

SOFT GLOW

A supremely relaxed everyday look: apricot blusher on the cheeks and shimmery eyes give Martina's face a youthful vibrancy – the kind of radiant beauty that usually comes from a stroll along the beach.

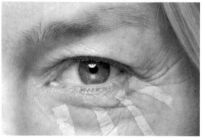

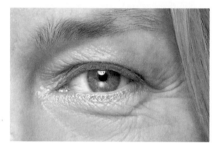

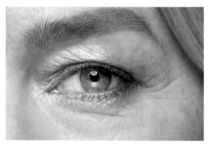

1 CONCEAL
Use concealer to disguise any small wrinkles and dark shadows around the eyes. Apply in a radial direction below the eye and then blend in gently using your finger.

2 HIGHLIGHT
Apply a nude-coloured, shimmery eyeshadow to the entire eyelid, extending above the crease, and blend in gently towards the outer corner of the eye.

3 EMPHASIZE
Fill in the eyebrows using a pale brown eyebrow powder. Define the outer corner of the eye using a darker colour, and apply plenty of mascara to the eyelashes.

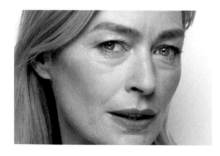

4 FINISHING TOUCHES
Apply apricot-coloured blusher generously to the cheekbones. Dab a bit of lip balm onto your lips and then colour them in using a lip liner pencil in a pale rosewood shade.

SOFT IS MORE YOUTHFUL

Softer lines for the eyebrows and eyes have a rejuvenating effect and make any wrinkles less noticeable. So, for the eyebrows, use a gently pigmented eyebrow powder or dot individual hairs with an eyebrow pencil rather than drawing a continuous line. For daytime make-up, use a soft kohl pencil around your eyes instead of a strong eyeliner; the effect can be softened even further by smudging with a foam applicator or cotton bud.

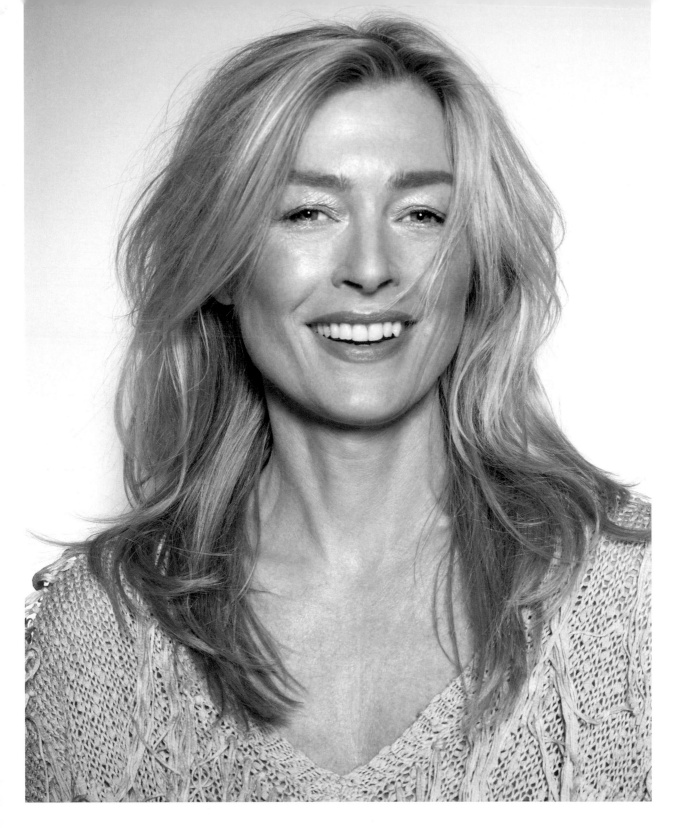

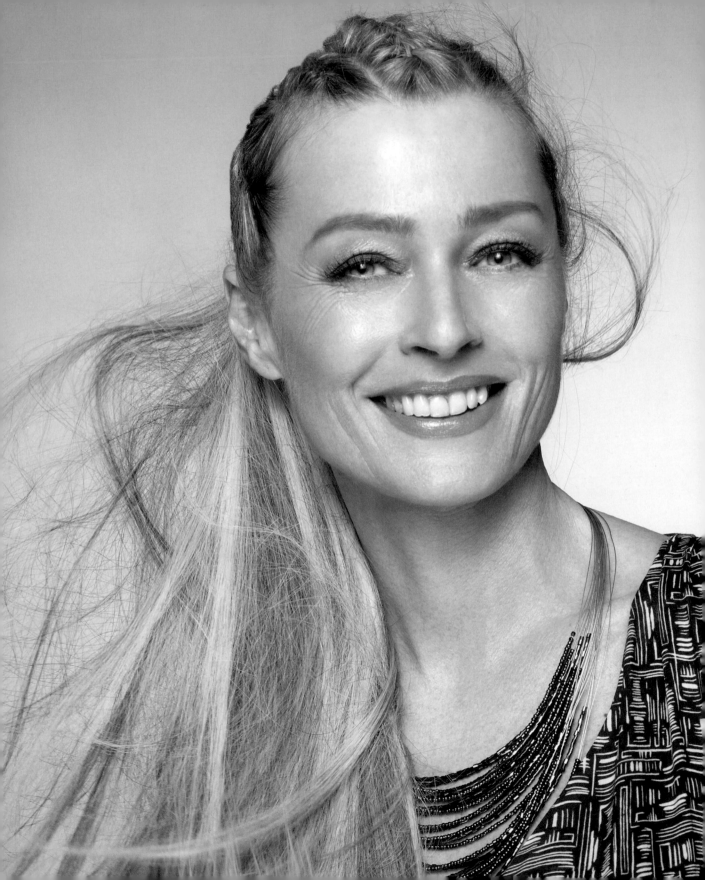

TIME OFF

A great look for the beach or for summer in the city. Martina has beautiful blue eyes with slightly droopy eyelids. A real eye-opening impact can be created using a shimmery eyeshadow, combined with strong eyebrows and a little cheating.

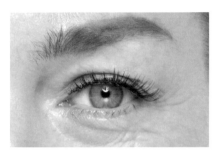

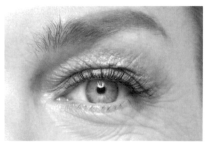

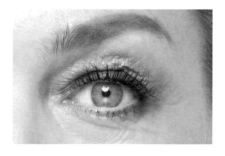

1 EMPHASIS
Emphasize the eyebrows using a pale brown eyebrow powder and shape them carefully. Curl the eyelashes and fill with individual false lashes and mascara.

2 SHADE
Use a brush to apply a silver-grey eyeshadow over the entire eyelid, and gently blend upwards, over the crease.

3 TRICKERY
Fix a magic strip (see p.12) into the eyelid crease. Add some gentle shading along the lash line and in the crease, using an anthracite-coloured eyeshadow.

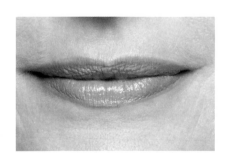

4 SCULPT
Carefully trace the contours of the lips using a nude lip liner and apply a pink-tinted lip gloss.

Where there are lots of fine lines around the eyes, concealer should not be too powdery. Lighter, more liquid concealers don't settle in the creases quite so readily.

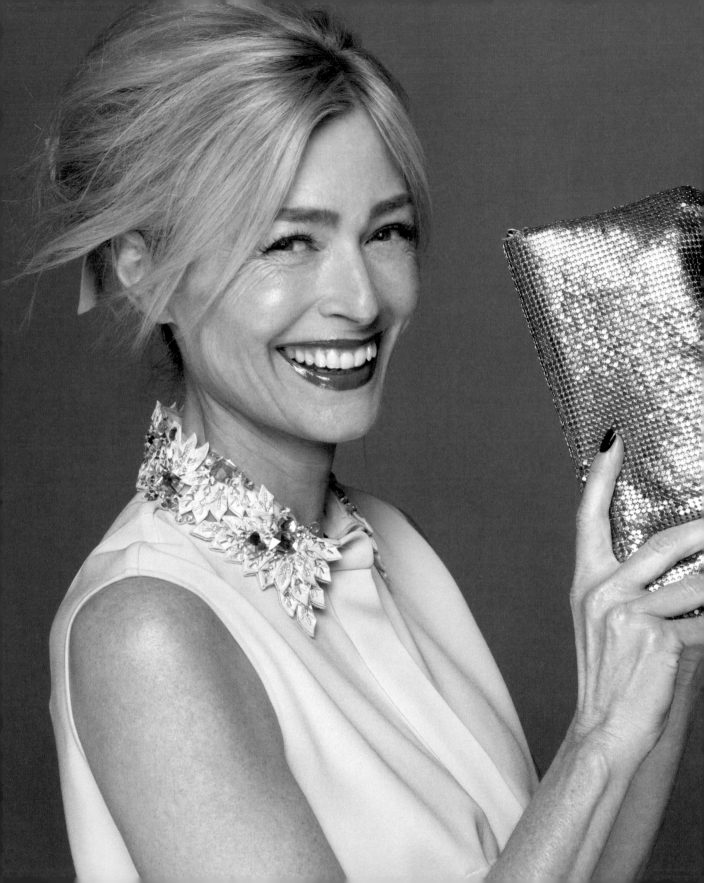

THINK PINK

For Martina I have conjured up an evening look that evokes rock 'n' roll, the twist, and circle skirts. The focus is on strong eyebrows, false eyelashes, and – for a particularly youthful look – deep pink lips.

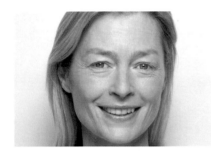 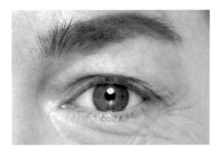 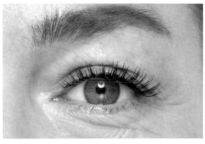

1 FOUNDATION
The ideal foundation, particularly for dry skin, is a moisturizing anti-ageing foundation with light-reflecting pigments. This will give your complexion a bright and fresh appearance.

2 EYEBROWS
Dot along the eyebrows using an eyebrow pencil or powder in a greyish brown shade, giving them a relatively broad shape, and fill in with the brush.

3 EYELASHES
Apply a neutral eyeshadow base to the eyelid. Apply mascara to the eyelashes and fix a strip of false lashes along the upper lash line of each eye using lash adhesive.

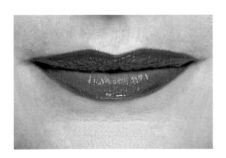

4 LIPS
Trace the outline of the lips using a pink lip liner and fill in, then apply pink lipstick. A dab of lip gloss in the centre gives the lips a fuller appearance.

Perfect lip contours: for a final touch, use some foundation on a small lip brush to neaten the contour of the lips from the outside.

LADIES NIGHT

Smoky eyes never go out of fashion. They can help make small eyes appear larger. In this special variant selected for Martina, the upper lid is dramatically emphasized, while the lower lash line gets just a subtle border.

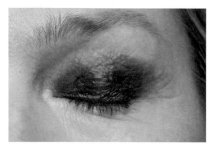

1 EYELIDS
Apply cream eyeshadow in a dark violet shade over the entire eyelid and just over the crease, blending with a brush.

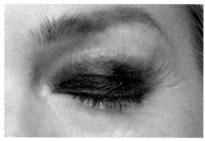

2 EYEBROWS
Set the eyeshadow by applying a thin layer of aubergine-coloured powder shadow. Fill in the eyebrows using a medium brown powder.

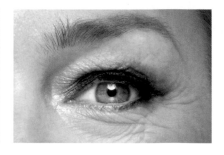

3 EYELASHES
Apply eyeliner to the upper lash line, and trace a thin line along the lower lashes; they should meet with an upward flick at the outer corner. Apply mascara generously.

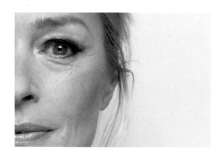

4 CHEEKS
Use a brush to apply peach powder blusher to the cheekbones and up to the temples, blending in gently.

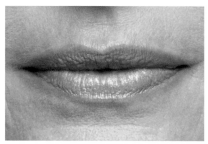

5 LIPS
Outline the lips with a pale pink lip liner, then apply a slightly pearlescent rose-coloured lipstick.

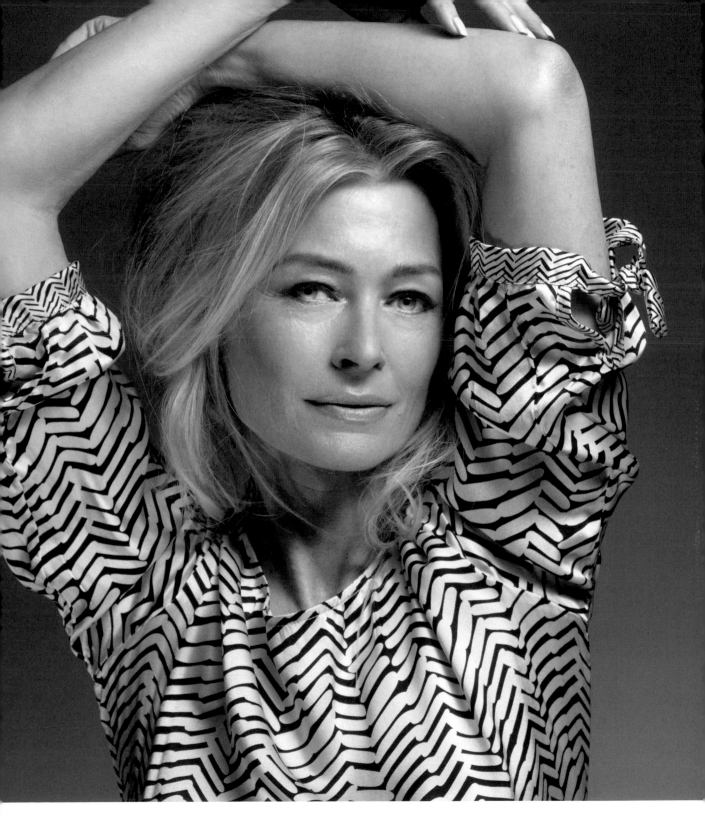

EYELASHES

Surely no other make-up product has such a stunning impact on your overall appearance as mascara. It can extend and thicken the lashes and provide volume. It also gives a whole new definition to the eyes.

A RANGE OF LOOKS

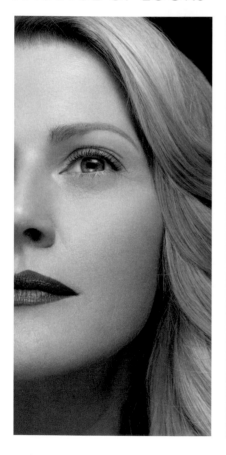 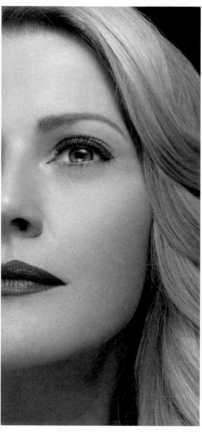 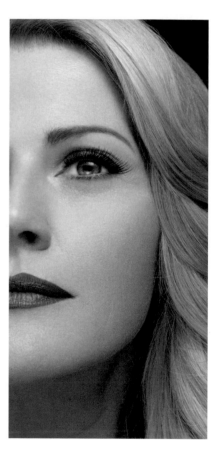

Soft: A basic mascara makes pale, delicate lashes immediately more visible. This emphasizes the eyes and opens them up.

Intense: A volume mascara coats each individual eyelash, making the lashes appear thicker. The important thing with mascara is to focus on the base of the lashes.

Dramatic: False eyelashes can be used to achieve a wide range of effects, from very natural to extravagant.

CURL

An eyelash curler is an invaluable tool when it comes to beautiful eyelashes, ensuring the lashes on the upper lid are more visible. It is not just for use on relatively short, straight lashes, but improves the curl on all types of lashes, with the result that they appear longer.

The classic eyelash curler is made of metal and has a silicon pad. Before purchase, make sure that the upper metal edge is rounded rather than sharp. This is how to use it: position your eyelashes close to the roots on the eyelash curler and squeeze together firmly for a few seconds. Then move the eyelash curler a couple of millimetres out from the eye and squeeze the eyelashes again. This helps give the lashes a perfect, natural curl.

COLOUR

After curling, it's time to deploy the mascara. There is a whole range of different types of brush, from thin to thick to curved, some with longer plastic bristles or shorter rubber ones. You will need to experiment to see which helps you achieve your desired effect. When applying mascara, it is best to start with the finest, shortest lashes at the upper inner corner of the eye, then work on the roots of the longer lashes at the outer corner. Always apply mascara to the base of the lashes first, ideally several applications. Only once you have done this should you apply mascara along the lengths of the lashes to the tips. This creates volume without clumping.

FALSE EFFECT

Wonderful effects can be created with false eyelashes. First, curl your own lashes upwards using an eyelash curler. Apply an extremely thin layer of rubber adhesive along the false eyelash strip and let it dry briefly. Then place the eyelash strip as close as possible to your upper lash line, and press it onto the skin. Look down and let the adhesive dry briefly. Then use mascara to blend your own eyelashes into the false lashes, working from the base up.

TIPS & TRICKS

Normally mascara is applied at the end, after eyeshadow and eyeliner. Here is a simple trick to prevent you getting little spots of mascara on your eye make-up: take a teaspoon with its curved back facing upwards and place it on the upper eyelid, moving it carefully upwards. Apply mascara over the back of the spoon – it works every time!

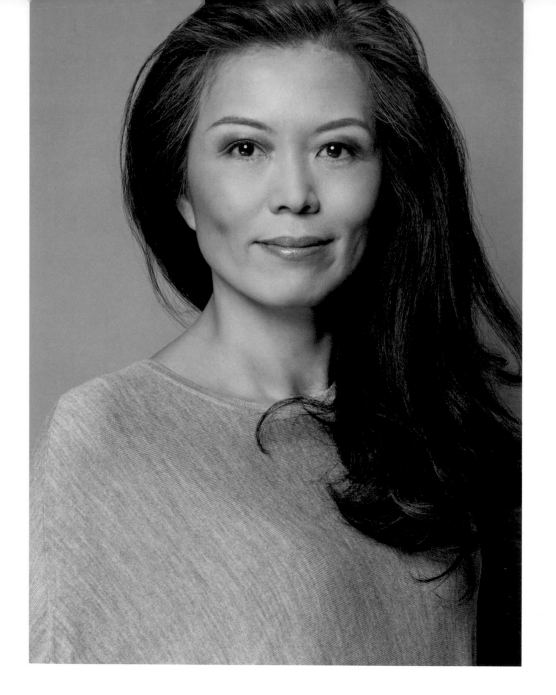

Highlights on the natural countours
of your face make you appear instantly
youthful and fresh-faced.

BRIGHT EYES

Would you like to lift drooping eyelids, hide dark shadows, and make your eyes truly shine? A touch of concealer in the right colours and glossy eyeshadow in warm shades will help you achieve this.

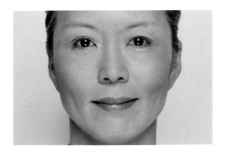

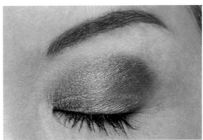

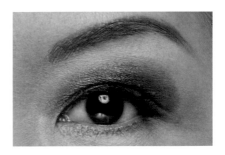

1 BASE

Apply foundation across the whole face to even out the skin tone. Use a concealer around the eyes to hide any dark circles. Blend in a contouring cream one shade darker right below the cheekbones.

2 EYES 1

Apply a dark eyeshadow to the eyelid, up to the crease. Fill the eyebrows with an eyebrow pencil and fix brows in place with a brow gel.

3 EYES 2

Apply a brown-gold eyeshadow into the crease and up towards the brow-bone. Apply mascara to the upper eyelashes only.

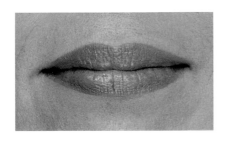

4 MOUTH

Outline the lips using a lip liner in the same colour as your natural lips, then fill in with a lipstick in the same colour. For a more natural effect, apply the lipstick using your finger.

WIDE-EYED

The characteristic Asian eyelid with no crease is known in the Asian region as a "single eyelid". The "double eyelid" (with crease), as is common in Western nations, makes the eye seem larger and the face seem more alert. With practice the crease can be defined through proper shading. A warm-gray or cool-brown work particularly well. Use an eyeshadow brush to apply the eyeshadow in small right-left movements from the inner to the outer corner of the eye when the eye is open.

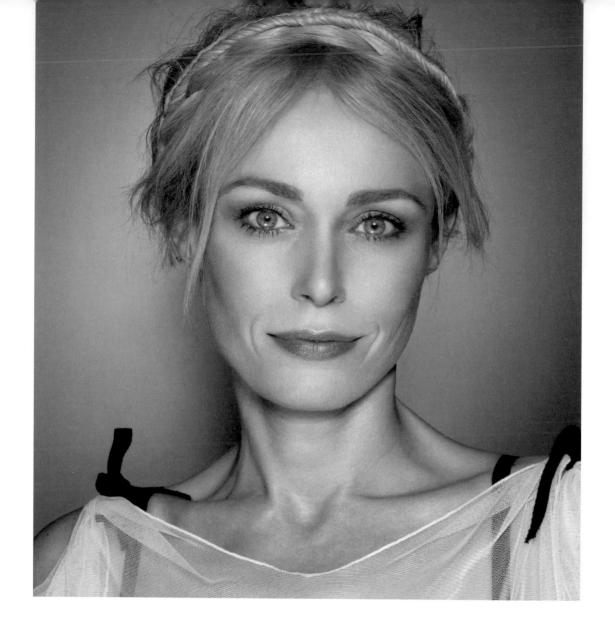

SIMPLY FABULOUS

Soft and romantic, Julia's look makes use of delicate colours that give her a fresh and radiant appearance.

Never test the colour of a concealer on the back of your hand – try it out on your face, where it belongs. The same goes for foundation.

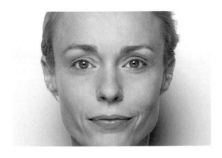

1 FOUNDATION

Carefully distribute foundation over the skin and gently blend outwards from the centre using your fingers. This helps create a smooth and radiant complexion.

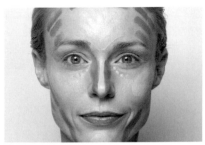

2 SCULPTING

Disguise any redness or under-eye shadows using a light concealer, then add some shading to the forehead, nose, and chin to create the effect of narrower contours.

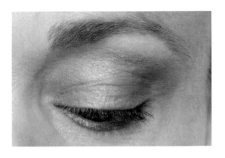

3 SHADING

Apply a pale pink satin eyeshadow over the entire eyelid, blending it out beyond the outer corner of the eye.

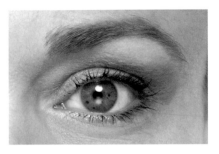

4 MASCARA

Apply mascara liberally to the eyelashes. Fill in any gaps in the eyebrows by dotting with an eyebrow pencil, and brush them into shape.

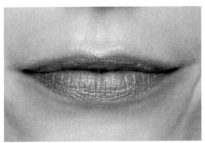

5 LIPS

Trace the outline of the lips with a pale lipliner and then apply a creamy coffee shade of lipstick, using a lip brush.

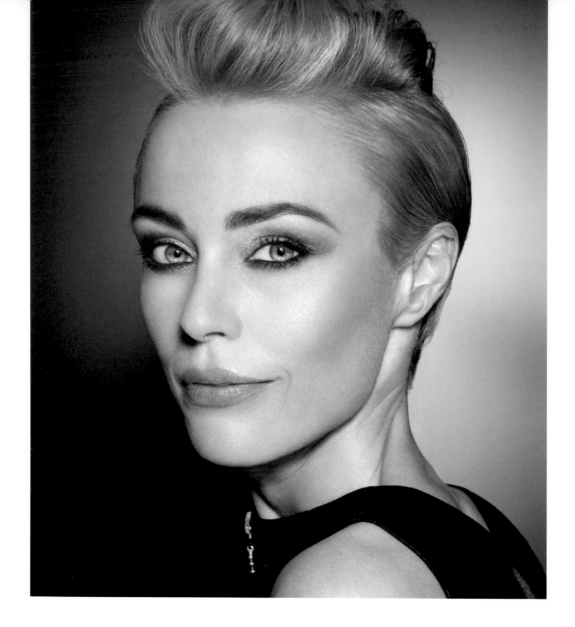

ROCK DELUXE

To go with Julia's short blonde hairstyle, I have selected make-up that really emphasizes her eyes. Giving the lips a nude look draws the focus of attention to the eye make-up.

An angular face will appear less severe if you apply darker foundation to the sides of the cheekbones down towards the chin and up to the temples.

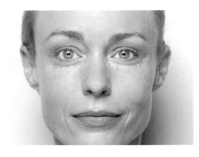

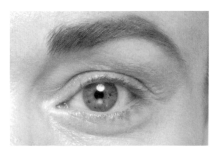

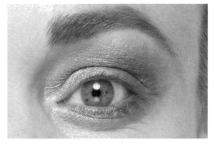

1 CONCEAL

Cover under-eye shadows using a concealer with a yellow-orange tint that matches the skin tone. Gently pat it into the skin with your finger.

2 FILL

Fill in missing hairs in the eyebrows using a medium brown eyebrow powder, then brush into shape.

3 FRAME

Apply a pink-gold shadow beyond the eyelid crease. Emphasize the outer corner and lower lash line in mauve. Add highlights to the inner corner and under the eyebrows with a pale colour.

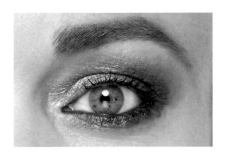

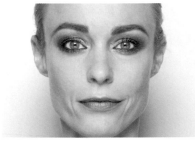

4 MASCARA

Add some shading to the eyelid crease and below the eye with a rust-coloured eyeshadow. Draw along the lower waterline with a black kohl eyeliner. Apply mascara liberally to the upper and lower lashes.

5 MOUTH

The lips can be left quite natural, with just a dab of gloss. For a more intense lip colour, use a nude shade of lipstick.

LIPS

A precise lip shape and well-chosen colour will distract from any minor wrinkles in the surrounding area. Your complexion will instantly appear fresher and your teeth will look whiter.

DEFINITION AND EMPHASIS

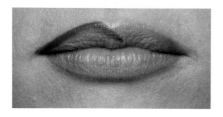 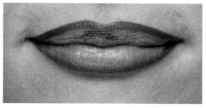 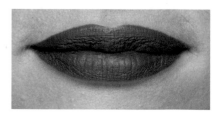

1 Outline the curve of the lips: Only a sharp lip liner will produce a neat line. Draw each half of the line in a single go from the corner of the mouth to the centre. Stretch the lips slightly while doing this.

2 Outline the lower lip: Take care when drawing the line along the lower lip that you can always see the tip of the lip liner.

3 Fill in the lips: Colour in the lips with the lip liner. Then use a lip brush to apply lipstick, keeping within the line.

TIPS & TRICKS

1. Less is more – and looks younger. A lip liner in a natural colour produces the best lip outline and shape, while ensuring the lipstick stays exactly where intended.
2. Instead of precisely painted lips, apply lip balm and dab on the lipstick using your finger. This helps make stronger colours look softer, or just gives the lips a natural, fresh appearance.
3. Ombré looks can make narrow lips appear larger. Colour in the lips entirely in one colour and then use your fingertip to dab on a darker shade in the centre of the lips.

CARE

Lip colours can only look their best if lips are well cared for. When you are brushing your teeth, run the toothbrush over your lips. This encourages the circulation and removes any little flakes of skin. When you perform your next facial scrub, include the lips too. As the seasons change, use a lip balm that contains natural plant waxes and oils. You can also buy special lip care creams, serums, and primers that nourish and smooth the skin on the lips, creating a perfect base for your lipstick.

COLOUR

When choosing a lipstick colour there are no rules or regulations, just a couple of recommendations. Women with a cool complexion and a reddish undertone will find that bluish colours, such as pink, violet, and berry tones, suit them particularly well. For women with a warm skin tone, shades with a yellowy component, such as apricot, terracotta, coral, or orange, are the most flattering. Very dark, strong lipstick shades make the mouth appear smaller, whereas paler, brighter colours make it appear larger.

VARIETY

Long-lasting lipsticks are ideal for more mature lips. They won't stray into any fine lines; instead, the colour stays right where it belongs. Coloured, delicately tinted or clear lip gloss applied to the centre of the lips has the effect of making them seem fuller.

LIPS WITH A GLOSS FINISH

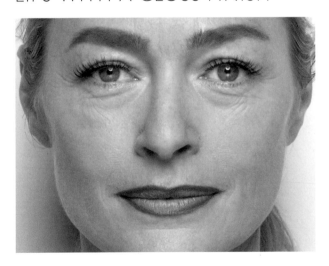

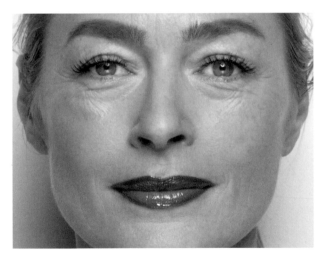

1 Contour: Apply a lip primer just as carefully as your lipstick. Then outline the lips using a lip liner as described, see left.

2 Colour and shine: Carefully colour the entire lips with the lip pencil, and dab clear or tinted lip gloss onto the lips.

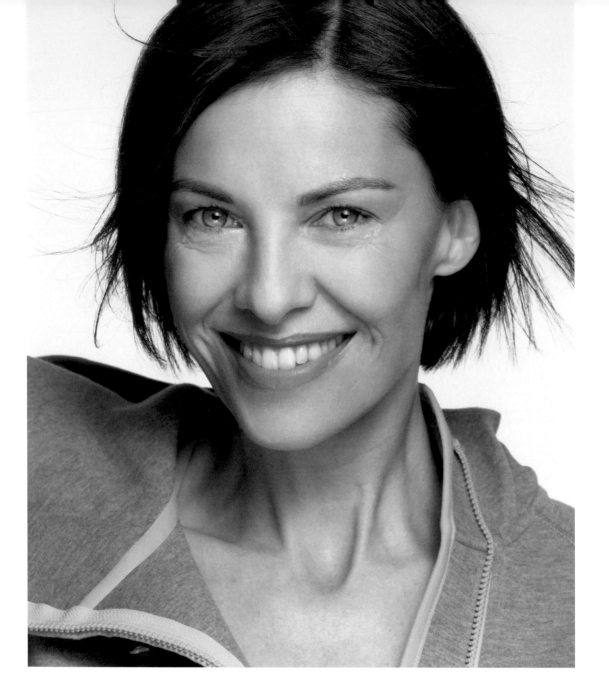

On your travels and forgotten your eyebrow pencil? A matte brown eyeshadow is great for filling in eyebrows.

SPORTY STYLE

A cosy weekend at home or a little time out at a spa hotel are both great occasions for this relaxed style, as modelled by Almuth. Eyes, lips, and complexion have a super fresh, sporty, and totally natural appearance.

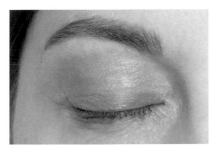 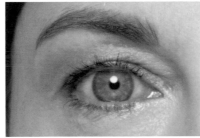 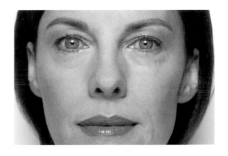

1 EYELIDS
Add emphasis to the eyelid with an all-over pale pink colour, and use a brush to softly shade up towards the brow bone.

2 EYELASHES
Curl the lashes using an eyelash curler and apply mascara. Fill in the eyebrows by gently dotting with a light brown eyebrow pencil.

3 FINISH
Add a bit of shading beneath the cheekbones and apply some pale pink blusher to the highest point of the cheekbones. Finish off with some peach lip gloss.

EXPRESS COMPLEXION

If you have to wear make-up all week long for work, it is nice to have a bit of time off at the weekend. But particularly for women who rarely spend time outside in their day-to-day life, the complexion can often appear washed-out without foundation. One solution is to try a self-tanning lotion. Recent formulas brighten up the skin tone in no time at all, without giving you an unattractive orange hue. What's more, they are often enriched with nourishing ingredients such as antioxidants and hyaluronic acid, so you can do without your moisturizing day cream.

FRESH & SMART

Perfect for work, a family do, or a trip to the theatre: Almuth's expressive eyes are enhanced by a diffused eye line created with soft black kohl. The lips are emphasized with a rosewood shade.

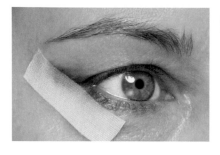

1 TAPING
A fantastic trick if you find it hard to pull off the cat flick freehand: stick on a piece of low-tack tape at an angle.

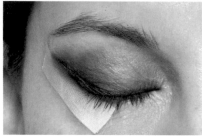

2 BLURRING
Use kohl to draw a line along the upper lash line. Use an eye shadow blender to shade the lid and eyeliner with a smoky eyeshadow.

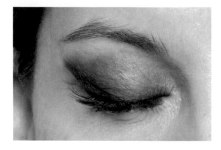

3 MASCARA
Curl the lashes with an eyelash curler and add some strong black volume mascara. Separate the lashes with an eyelash brush.

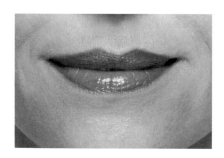

4 LIPS
Outline the lips with a lip liner pencil, apply lipstick in a creamy berry shade, and dab on some gloss with your finger.

PHOTO FINISH

Do you always look slightly shiny in photographs? It could be that you've overdone it with the moisturizer. Normally a well-moisturized complexion looks fantastic, but in photographs this glow can often look greasy. So, before you have the next shot taken for the family album, dab your T-zone area with some oil-control facial blotting paper, or use a touch of loose or pressed translucent powder.

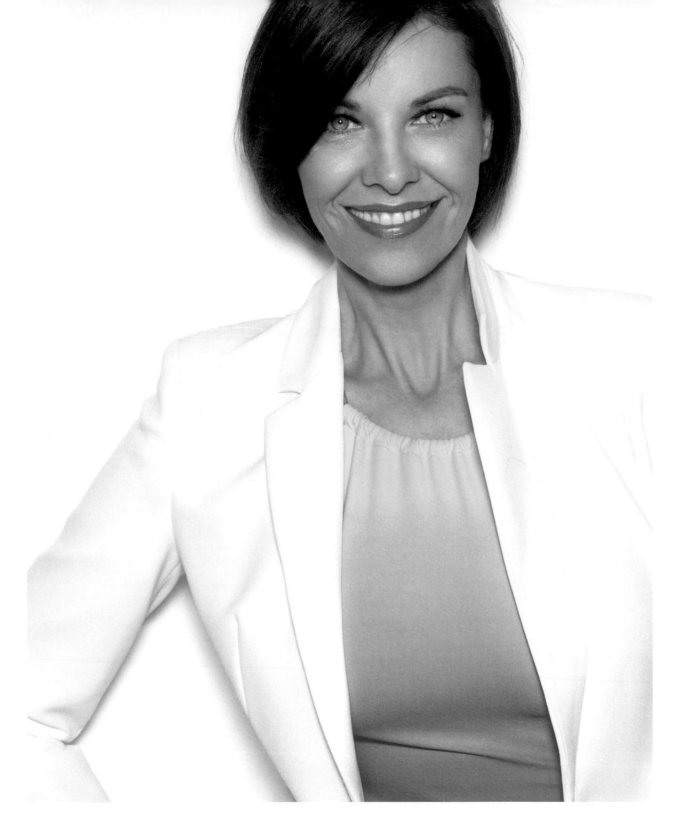

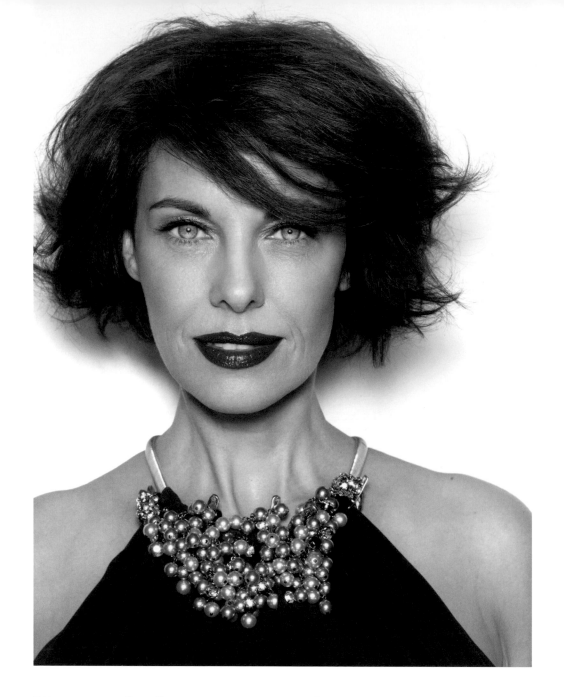

Nervous before your grand entrance? Spritz a little thermal water onto your skin; this reduces any irritation and helps your make-up last longer.

OUTGOING

A great look for a stylish party or an elegant dinner: Almuth's lips shine in a rich, warm red colour, and her blue-green eyes sparkle, enhanced by a high-shimmer deep pink shade.

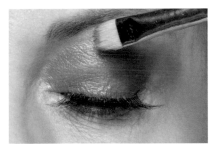

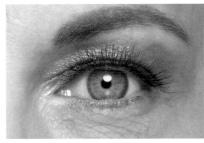

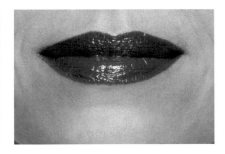

1 LIDS
Apply a base layer of eye primer over the entire lid and leave it to set. Then apply a pink shade of eyeshadow and blend it out over the eyelid crease.

2 EYELASHES
Apply mascara liberally, not forgetting the fine lashes at the inner and outer corners of the eyes. Fill in the eyebrows using a brow powder and brush them into shape.

3 MOUTH
Outline the lips using a lip liner pencil and then carefully apply a warm red lipstick using a lip brush.

A QUICK COVER-UP

Of course, spots always appear just before a particularly important event … but you can banish these troublemakers for the evening. Use a concealer brush to pick up a bit of creamy concealer in a colour that exactly matches your skin tone. Brush this gently over the blemish, and then press it into the skin with a gently rolling finger movement until the colour virtually blends into the surrounding skin. Don't rub, or you will just remove most of the concealer again.

"Yes, we can!"

Nothing ever stands still in Eveline Hall's life: she needs a constant buzz and is always on the search for new experiences. Her motto is: never give up – and constantly reinvent yourself, even in old age.

Eveline Hall arrives at the photo studio – slim and tall, in black drainpipe trousers, suede boots, and leather jacket, radiating so much energy, the sparks are flying! There is no doubt she makes her presence felt. But Eveline Hall is no capricious diva. She comes across as unpretentious, straightforward, honest, and highly pragmatic. The daughter of a prima ballerina and an actor, Eveline was born in Greifswald and grew up in Hamburg. She has had all sorts of jobs and can look back on a very varied career. She first danced at the Hamburg State Opera House, then in the 1970s she was a showgirl in Paris and Las Vegas, and later worked as a stage actress in Hamburg, Basel, Munich, and Strasbourg. She married an American, but was divorced after nine years. She fell in love with a Frenchman and lives in Paris.

"Every so often I need to have a fresh start"

At one point, Eveline was drawn back to her native Hamburg, partly to be closer to her mother. At a time when others are reminiscing about middle age or are contemplating acquiring a caravan, Eveline is still exploring and challenging herself. She offers personal training, presents fashion shows at trade fairs, films small commercials – and makes a good living from all these activities. But curiosity and ambition drive her onwards: she's taking singing lessons, she studies texts following her own methodology, and she has developed a power ballet workout for herself and her mother, which they complete on a daily basis.

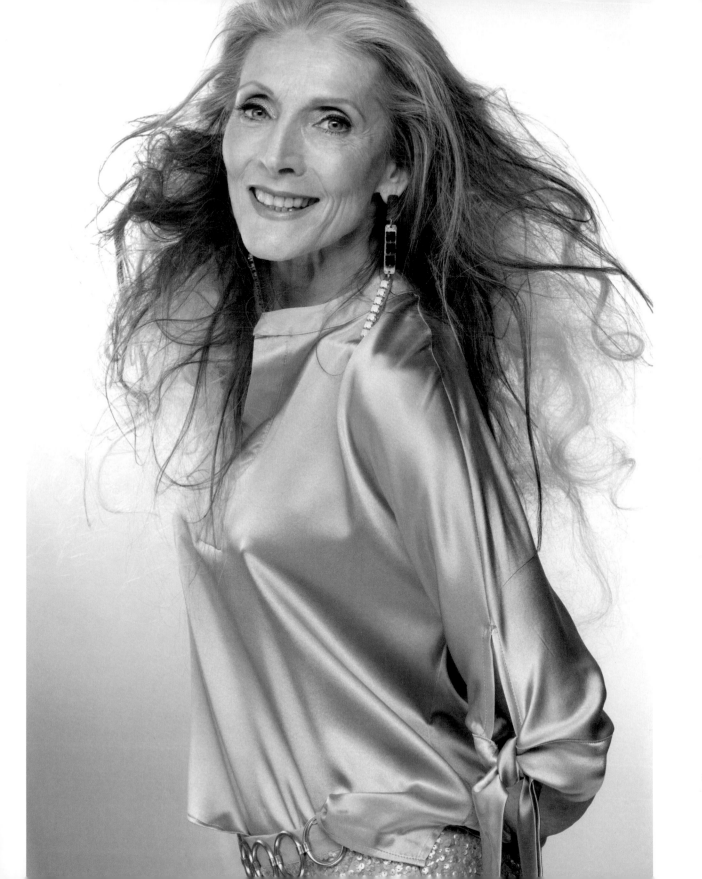

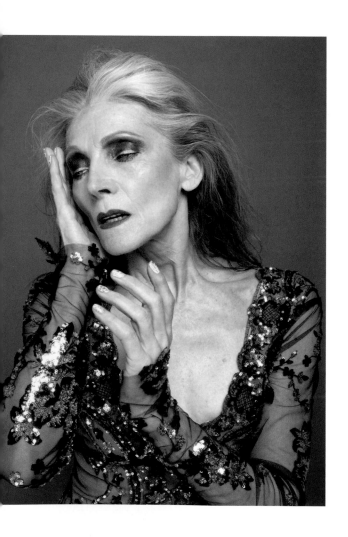

Her career as a model didn't even kick off until she was 65. Following advice from a good friend, Eveline applied to a modelling agency that was not looking for young, pretty models, but wanted real people for their advertisements. She was accepted and, soon afterwards, found herself on set for a well-paid commercial in Kiev. Photo shoots for cars and magazine spreads for the likes of *GQ* soon followed. A highlight of her new career was shooting with famous photographer Ellen von Unwerth for a hair care product company. Originally, Eveline was intended to be a kind of "grandmother model" for the shoot, but before they knew it she was draping herself in a size 8 latex suit among top young models such as Coco Rocha and Lydia Hearst.

At the Berlin Fashion Week, she once again worked alongside young models – such as Toni Garrn at a show by Michalsky – and had lots of fun doing it. "The modelling world is just adorable. In the acting and dance scenes there is much more scheming," she says. But she still views the whole thing with a sense of perspective and humour: "To be modelling at my age is really a bit preposterous. I would never have had the idea of mixing with 15- to 20-year-olds. That was my agent's idea!"

"I'm just a happy person"

Anyway, classifications such as "silver generation" or "golden girl" are alien to Eveline Hall. She is not the type to be cultivating a rose garden at home or holidaying at a wellness retreat in a 5-star Bali resort. "I don't need all that. I'm just a happy person and I work a lot, exactly as I always have done."

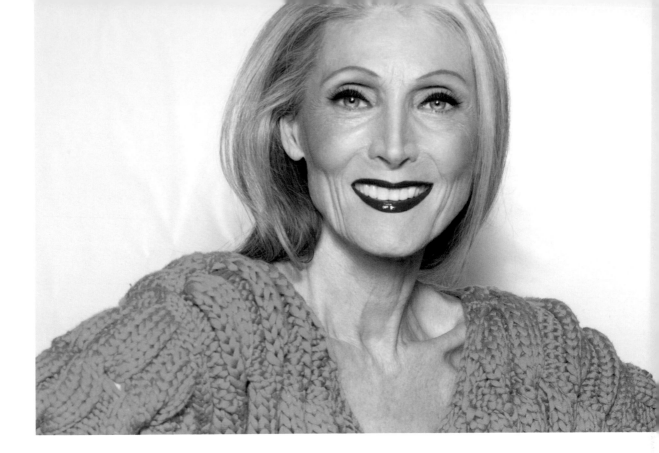

Eveline looks great, but not "young for her age". Perhaps the reason for this is that she rejects artificial beauty. Her hair has not been dyed for a long time and she just uses a simple cream to care for her skin. She regards cosmetic surgery as simply absurd. Her aesthetic ideals are represented by women like Meryl Streep. "Or also Judi Dench – what a great lady," says Eveline.

She finds the question about being afraid of ageing pretty foolish – would she be sitting here if she was? Her only fear is of illness. And above all, perhaps, not being able to stop at the right time. In her book *Stepping out and putting on my own show* she concludes: "It would be terrible if one day people were whispering 'here comes the old lady again.'" But Eveline is not thinking about stopping just yet. She has recently recorded a CD. "Every so often you need to give your brain a challenge and have some imagination" – a motto that also represents her approach to life. Without doubt, it can be ours too.

FASHIONABLY GREY

Not so long ago, grey hair was inseparable from retirement and old age, but nowadays it is very much in vogue. There's no doubt that grey hair can look gorgeous – here's some advice to help make the most of it.

WHY DOES HAIR GO GREY?

Grey hair does not really exist. It is in fact unpigmented and therefore white. The impression of greyness arises from the interplay between these white hairs and the remaining coloured hair. Our hair loses colour over time because the body produces less tyrosine. This amino acid is responsible for creating the hair and skin pigment melanin. Most people initially begin to go grey at the hairline and the temples.

FROM COLOUR TO SILVER

When the first grey hairs appear as fine strands of silver at the roots, they are not very noticeable. But as the hair continues to grow and the grey hairs multiply, at some point you have to decide: artificial colour or go properly grey. The transition from colour to grey can be made easier by getting ultrafine highlights put in by an expert stylist. Don't try to dye your hair completely grey, as this looks unnatural (a helmet effect) and it will make you look much older. Women with blonde hair often have to cope with an unattractive yellowy tint as they go grey. This can be balanced out by using a bluey-violet colour shampoo and conditioner. Not everyone goes grey evenly. If the proportion of white and still pigmented hair looks too pallid, dyeing the hair blonde can help achieve a more radiant colour and looks more youthful than grey hair.

A GLOSSIER GREY

Grey hair is structurally quite different to pigmented hair. It seems tougher and thicker, it sometimes goes frizzy and is brittle. That is why it is important to use anti-ageing hair care products that are specially designed for grey hair. These contain intensely nourishing ingredients from plant oils along with ceramides and proteins that smooth out the cuticle layer, add gloss, and at the same time have a gently straightening effect on unruly hair. Similarly, with styling products you should opt for smoothing products, such as wax and finishing creams. As you blow-dry, comb the hair through with your fingers, and then finish by blow-drying over a round brush. This gives the hair lots of body.

THE BEST HAIRCUT

The softer and more flowing the haircut, the fresher and more natural it will appear. A fringe and/or strands that fall slightly over the face draw attention to the more animated eye area. Volume at the roots flatters the facial structure. Fashionable haircuts, such as geometric bobs, pixie cuts, and other short styles can look great, but be careful: these need to fit in to an "overall look", that is to say, they need appropriate make-up and styling for maximum impact. Of course, grey hair can also be worn long.

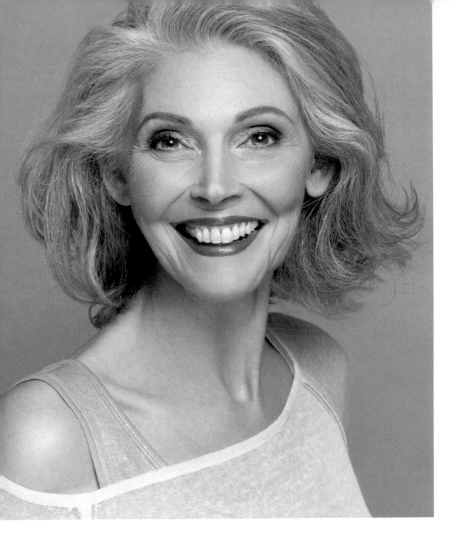

Varying shades of silver in the hair appear more vibrant than a uniform grey.

PERFECT MAKE-UP FOR GREY HAIR

Grey hair requires contrast to avoid the complexion appearing tired, sallow, or too pale. Lips in apricot, coral, or delicate shades of pink work well. For the eyelids, shimmery gold or silver, and shades of green or grey work perfectly. Blusher is nearly always essential with grey hair. Here too it is best to select fresh, natural shades such as peach or pink, rather than terracotta or brown. Statement nails are a fantastic partner for grey hair: in hot pink, bold red, jazzy orange, or deep magenta.

ETERNAL BEAUTY

For Barbara, I have selected colours to go with her grey hair that make her fair complexion look younger, more expressive, but very natural. The focus is on subtly emphasized eyes and — importantly — some blusher for added radiance.

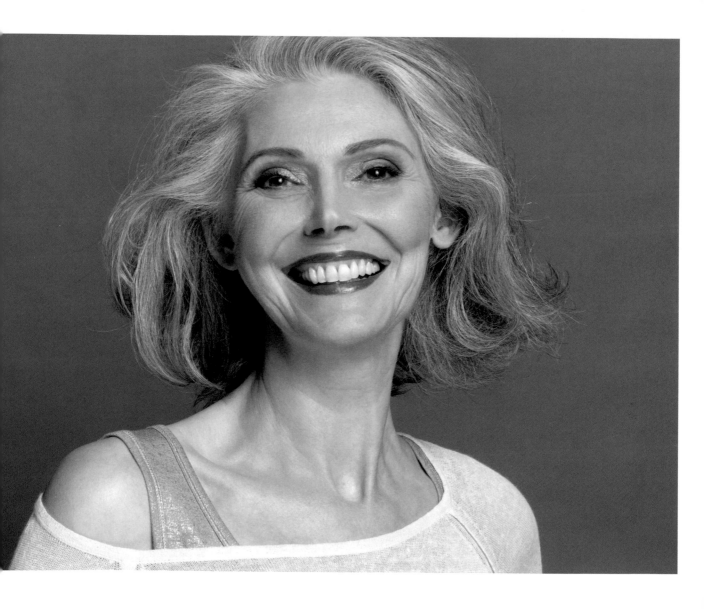

Particularly with grey hair, look out for expressive, flattering lipstick colours. Vivid nude shades and more intense berry and coral tones are just the thing.

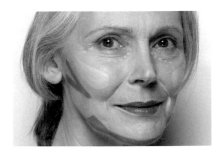

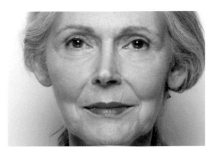

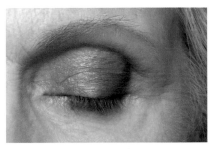

1 CONTOURING
Use a moisturizing anti-ageing foundation with soft-focus pigments. Cover any under-eye shadows or red areas with concealer, and add some shading.

2 BLENDING
Gently blend highlights and shading with your fingers. The shading sharpens facial contours and helps the cheekbones stand out, while the highlights emphasize other areas.

3 EYE SHADOW
Apply a pale brown shimmer eyeshadow over the eyelid, adding a darker brown shade from the outer corner of the eye to the crease.

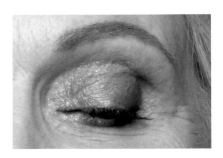

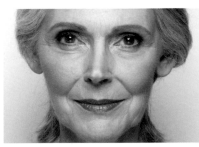

4 HIGHLIGHTS
Pale nude highlights at the inner corner of the eye open up the eyes and make them look more alert. Fill in the eyebrows subtly using a brow powder.

5 BLUSHER
Apply a delicate apricot powder blusher from the cheeks up to the temples using a brush, and blend in gently.

FRESH FACE

Bronze shades work amazingly well with grey hair, giving a fresh, revitalized feel. The key is to combine them with a vibrant lipstick in a strong coral shade.

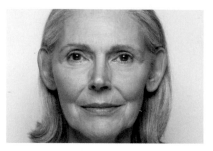

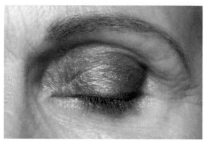

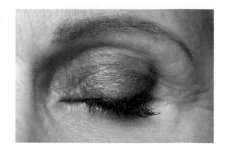

1 FOUNDATION

Apply liquid foundation to the face and leave to set briefly. Use a blusher brush to apply bronzing powder to the high points of the face.

2 EYE SHADOW

Apply a bronze eyeshadow to the entire eyelid and over the crease, blending in softly with a lighter gold shade.

3 EYELINER

Draw a line using brown kohl along the upper lash line and smudge with a blender brush. Apply plenty of mascara to the eyelashes.

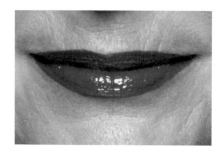

4 LIPSTICK

Outline the lips with a coral-coloured lip liner and then fill them in. Apply a glossy lipstick on top.

LIP BOOSTER

Over the course of time, most women's lips become thinner, because they are no longer producing as much collagen, which is needed to ensure plump lips and smooth skin. There is a solution: skilful use of lip liner to produce the best lip shape and sharpen up the lip contours. Also make sure you use creamy, ideally semi-transparent, glossy lipsticks. These make the lips look plumper. A specialized lip cream can also be used to smooth out fine lines around the mouth.

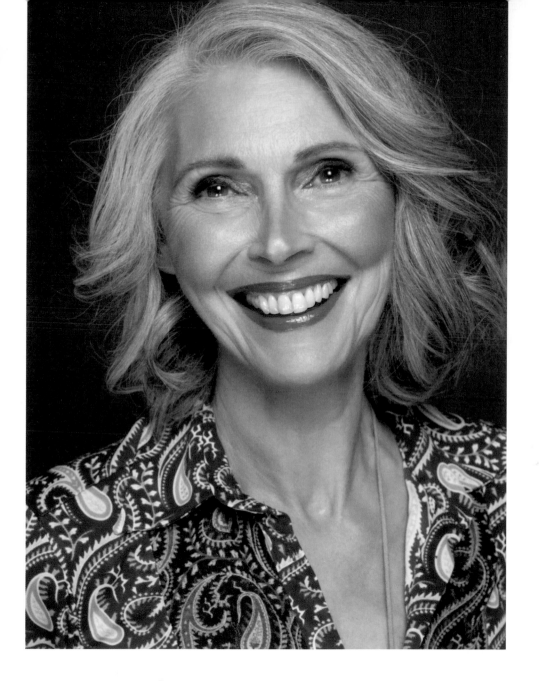

For Barbara's pale skin, the bronzer should be neither too orange nor too brown. Here, a subtle shade with cool undertones looks particularly natural.

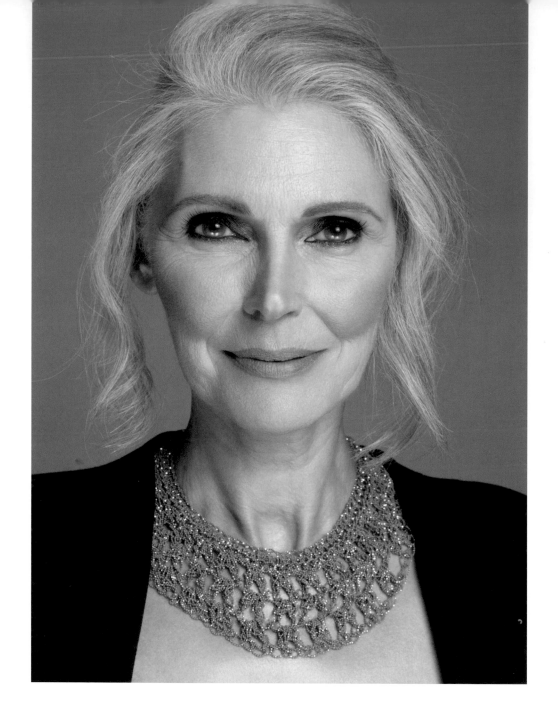

Some loose highlighter powder on the face, throat, and neckline provides additional glow.

ALL EYES ON ME

Barbara normally goes for a very natural look, but she wanted dramatic make-up for a special evening. Dark, shimmery eyeshadows in silver and black give this look a real wow factor.

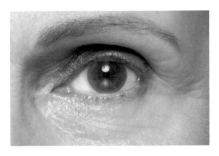

1 EYES 1

Apply silvery grey eyeshadow over the whole eyelid and blend softly outwards beyond the eyelid crease.

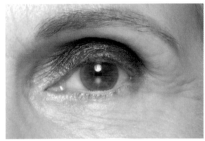

2 EYES 2

Blend in a black eyeshadow so that you get a straight vertical line at the outer corner of the eye. This gives the look a strong, modern appeal.

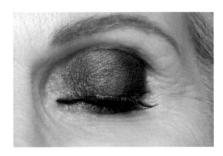

3 EYES 3

Use black kohl to draw a line along the eyelid at the upper lash line and along the lower waterline. Add shading with a grey eyeshadow to the lower lash line. Apply mascara liberally to the eyelashes.

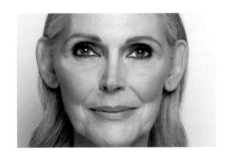

4 FINISH

Apply a peach blusher to the cheekbones. Finish with a creamy lipstick in a strong nude shade.

LOOKS FROM 1001 NIGHTS

In oriental countries real kohl is not only used as a cosmetic, but also to protect the eyes. In these countries, kohl pencils often have some camphor mixed in, which is supposed to be good for dry eyes. There is no question kohl is great for adding eye definition for the 40+ woman, and it lends a dramatic air, particularly when applied traditionally along the waterline on the lower and upper eyelids.

MAKE-UP WITH GLASSES

Glasses are a great fashion accessory that can be used to complete or transform a look in an instant. But if you wear glasses, what is the best way to wear make-up?

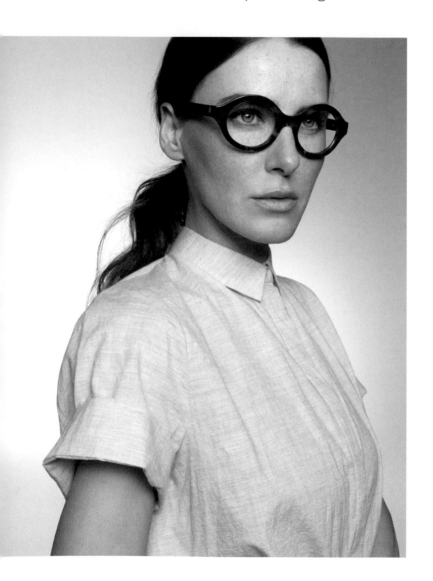

TIPS & TRICKS

Concealer is particularly important if you wear glasses. The frame and lens inevitably cast shadows onto the face and therefore under the eyes, so you can easily look tired. Here's the answer: apply your concealer in a fan shape under the eyes and extend it a bit lower down than usual – ideally down to the lower rim of the glasses frame.

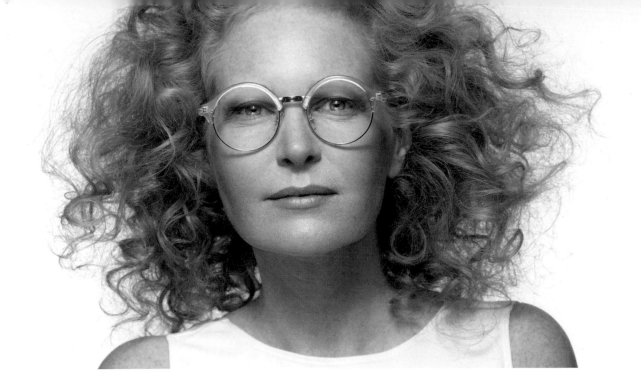

FOR THE SHORT-SIGHTED

Lenses that correct short-sightedness can make the eyes appear smaller. Pale, shimmery eye shadow on the eyelid and a darker shaded crease are the perfect eye-openers. It's also important to use plenty of mascara and an eyelash curler to open up the eyes.

If the eyes are close together, emphasize the outer part with a darker colour, then dab a pale metallic shadow at the inner corner of the eye. Be careful with dark kohl, as this can make the eyes seem smaller. Along the lower lash line, it is better to use a silver- or beige-coloured kohl; this makes the eyes appear larger and brighter.

FOR THE FAR-SIGHTED

The lenses used to correct far-sightedness have an effect rather like a magnifying glass: they make the eyes appear larger. That sounds like a good thing, but it also draws attention to any fine lines or under-eye shadows. Eye shadows that are matte or have a very subtle shimmer, in smoky tones such as grey-blue, mauve, or anthracite, are ideal for the far-sighted, since they emphasize the eyes without further enlarging them.

Lines drawn with eyeliner or kohl should always be very fine and softly diffused, since strong, harsh lines are also exaggerated through the lens of the glasses. Check your mascara application with a magnifying mirror, to make sure there is no clumping. Ideally, separate the lashes with a clean mascara brush after applying mascara.

STYLE & COLOUR

Depending on the style of your glasses, different features should be emphasized. With large, modern, wide-framed glasses, like those worn by Carolina (left), very little make-up is required; the lips should be given more emphasis than the eyes. If your make-up is too strong, it competes with the glasses and can end up making the whole eye area appear too dark. With large glasses, your eyebrows should either run parallel to the frame or, at most, extend very slightly above it.

With pale or rimless glasses, like those worn by Marion (above), the eyebrows need to be well shaped. Since these glasses are very neutral, your eye make-up can range from subtle to intense.

COPPER SHADES

Enviably, Marion has naturally curly red hair and sparkling green eyes. The main aim with this look is not to distract from her natural beauty, but to subtly enhance her complexion, eyes, and lips.

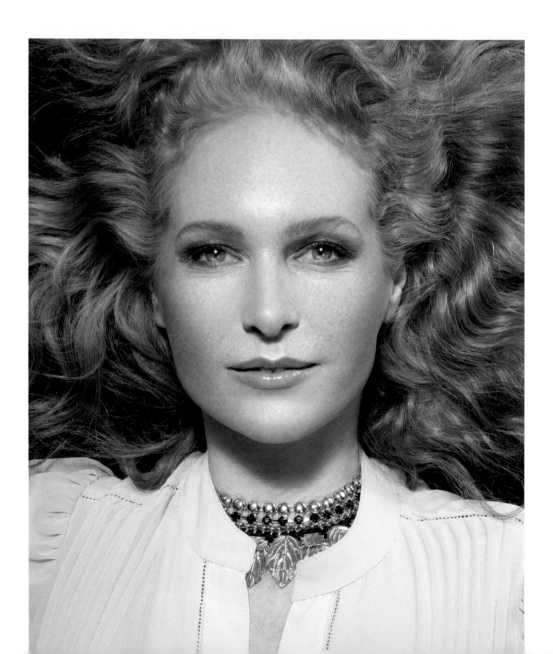

Where skin is pale and translucent, any bluish shadows under the eyes are best disguised using a concealer with a pale pink undertone.

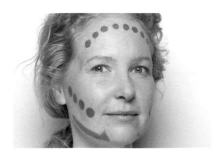

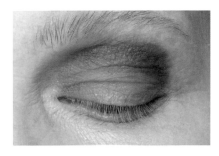

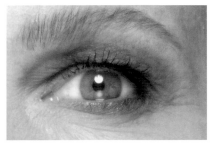

1 CONTOUR
Carefully apply foundation. Shading on the forehead makes it appear shorter. If used on the chin and cheek areas, it can make a rounder face appear more oval.

2 SHADE
Apply a pale pink eyeshadow to the entire eyelid and then blend into a golden brown colour in the crease.

3 EMPHASIZE
Fill in the eyebrows using a pale brown brow powder and shape using an eyebrow brush. Apply mascara just to the upper lashes.

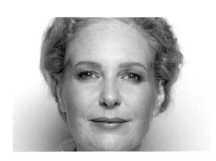

4 RADIANCE
Apply an apricot-coloured blusher to the front of the cheeks, then shade under the cheekbones using a bronzer. Intensify the natural lip colour using a gloss lipstick.

DOT TO DOT

Freckles should never be hidden under a thick covering of make-up. They will show through anyway, often appearing an unsightly shade of grey. A freckly complexion looks far more appealing when a transparent foundation, BB cream, or tinted moisturizer is used. Any small blemishes or red spots can be selectively masked with concealer.

MAGIC EYES

If there's one eyeshadow colour that red-haired women should get to know, it's green, in all its many and varied shades. Don't worry, when combined with otherwise subtle make-up, this look can be simply captivating.

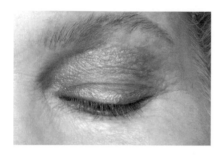 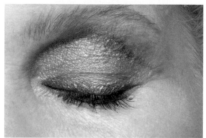 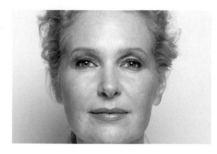

1 FOUNDATION
Apply a shimmer eyeshadow in an intense shade of green to the entire eyelid, extending over the crease.

2 SHADING
Apply a glittering gold eyeshadow over the green colour, adding emphasis with a warm brown shade on the brow bone.

3 FINISHING
Draw a line along the lower lash line using sea-green kohl and apply mascara to the lashes. Balance out the shape of the lips using a lip liner, and then apply gloss to accentuate.

A DELICATE AFFAIR

Red-haired women often have very pale and delicate eyelashes and eyebrows. To give them more impact you can either have them professionally coloured regularly or dye them yourself. Be very careful to get the colour right. Black and dark brown are far too dark for the eyebrows. A cool, light shade of brown is perfect. For the eyelashes, a blue-black, black, or more subtle dark brown are the best options. There are eyelash and eyebrow colours that are specifically designed for women with blonde or red hair. These shades tend to be called "natural", "light brown", and "blonde". Be sure to follow the instructions carefully so that the colour doesn't irritate the sensitive skin in this area.

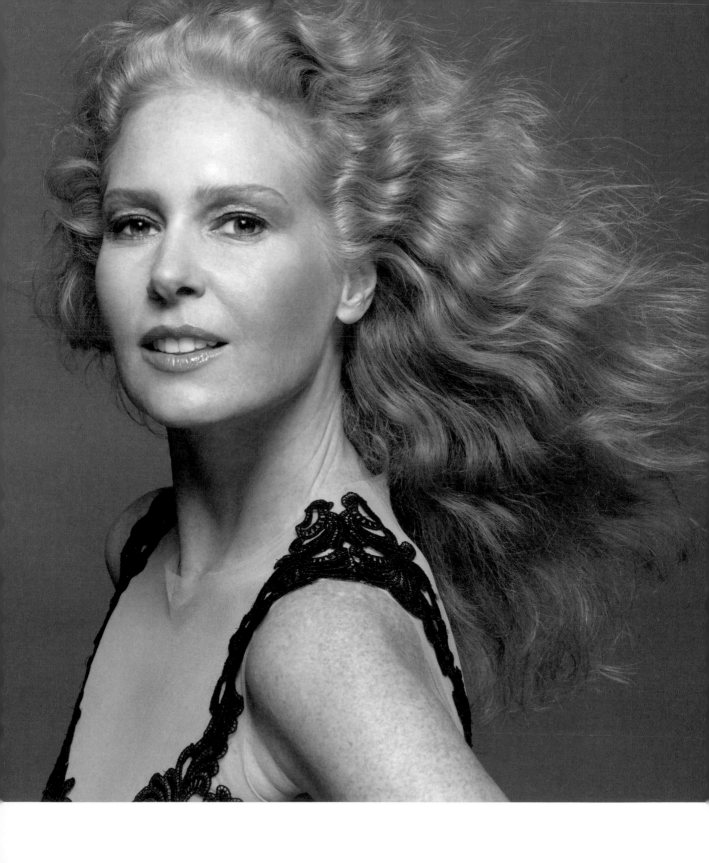

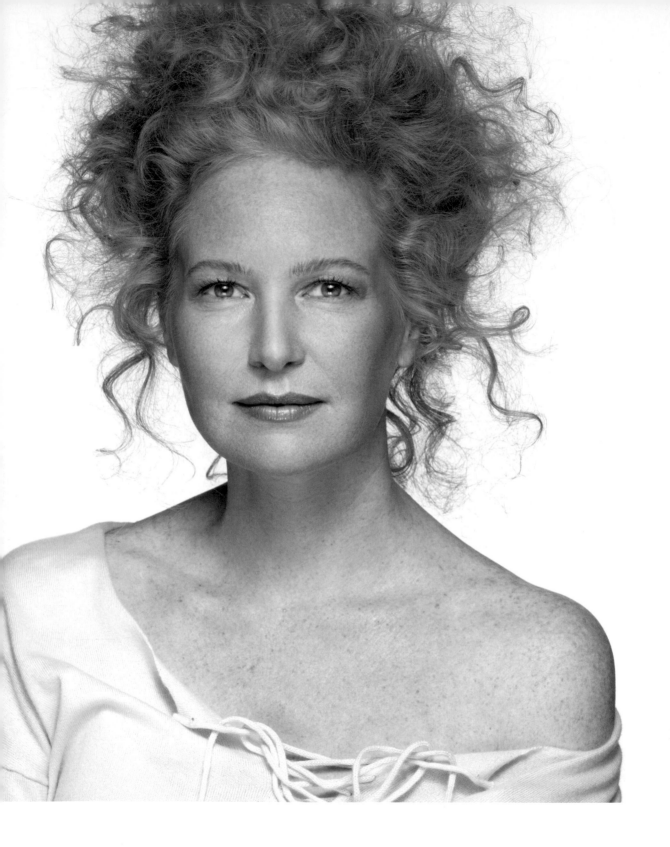

DESERT ROSE

The surprising thing about Marion's look is that a pink eyeshadow goes so superbly well with her red hair. It also combines beautifully with the warm terracotta on her lips and cheekbones.

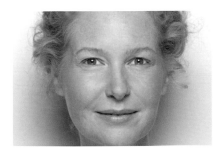

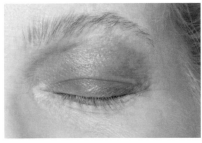

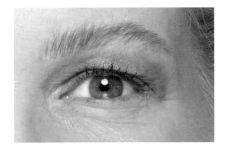

1 COMPLEXION
Even out the skin tone using a tinted moisturizer or a light, transparent foundation. This gives the complexion a delicate, natural appearance.

2 EYELIDS
Cover the entire eyelid with a pink eyeshadow and blend up towards the brow with a brush.

3 EYEBROWS
Trace the eyebrows with a light brown brow powder and apply several coats of mascara to the eyelashes.

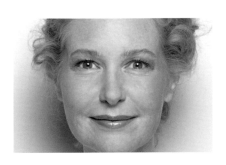

4 FINISH
Apply a subtle bronzer to the cheek area. Colour the lips with a terracotta shade of glossy lipstick.

To ensure that Marion's eyes look natural and subtle, I have consciously avoided circling them with eyeliner or kohl.

SOS TIPS FOR BEAUTY EMERGENCIES

With make-up, you're bound to make a mistake precisely when you're running late, and a spot is destined to appear just when you need it least. The following tips will save you from having a nervous breakdown.

WHAT CAN I DO IF ...

... I have dark shadows under my eyes in the morning? Use a concealer in a yellow/orange-tinted shade. This conceals the bluish discolouration caused by visible veins better than a concealer with a pink tone.

... I sneezed after applying mascara and now it has smeared under my eyes? Dip a cotton bud into an oil-free make-up remover and gently wipe away the little flecks. With the smoky eye look the mistake can quickly just be blended in.

... my hair is flat in the morning? There are special volume powders that include resins, which can be dusted carefully into the roots of the hair. By massaging in the powder, you prevent the hairs from lying quite so smoothly on top of each other, which creates a volumized effect.

... my lipstick has bled into the little lines and wrinkles around my mouth and now the outline is blurred? Smooth the skin around your lips with a special eye or lip care cream or with a lip primer, and use a lip pencil. Nowadays you can get transparent lip liners that go with any colour. The lip liner forms a barrier between the red and white areas on the lip skin. Long-lasting lipsticks are also less likely to bleed.

... an enormous spot has popped up on my chin this morning? Use a spot treatment with salicylic acid; this is the best way to ease inflammation and reduce redness. Conceal using a special cover stick or concealer.

... my cheeks suddenly start to "glow" during an important meeting? If you are susceptible to getting red cheeks, this is usually a sign that you have a reddish skin undertone. This can be balanced out by using a cool shade of foundation and a cool or even a green-tinted concealer. Dab an additional thin layer of concealer onto the most intensely reddened areas.

... my eyes are red? Eye drops with hyaluronic acid or eyebright can alleviate the problem. An optical trick is to apply a pale beige-coloured (not white!) kohl along the waterline of the lower eyelid. This helps balance out any redness visually.

... my cuticles are rough and ragged? Massage in pure shea butter every night before you go to sleep. This is absolutely the best and most intensive cuticle care product there is.

... my eyeshadow has settled into the little creases on my eyelid? Move your finger in a gentle circular direction over the eyelid, spreading the eyeshadow out again. Avoid this by using an eye primer with powder or cream eyeshadows.

... my dark nail varnish starts to chip on day two?
Add an overcoat. After drying apply a layer of top coat or clear varnish. If the varnish is seriously chipped, there's only one thing for it: take it all off with nail varnish remover and start again; anything else looks shabby, especially with dark nail polish shades.

... the delicate skin under my eyes is prone to puffiness? Hold two chilled tablespoons on the affected area for 5 minutes, or briefly put two used green tea teabags into the freezer and lay these on the closed eyelids for 5 minutes. The cold causes the blood vessels to contract and the swelling will reduce.

... my complexion is unattractively shiny just half an hour after doing my make-up? Beware of using too many layers of powder over the course of the day, as this can easily create a mask-like appearance. It's better to use oil-control facial blotting papers. These are wafer-thin sheets that soak up sebum (oily secretions) and so gently reduce any shininess. It is possible that your daily skin care cream is too rich.

... my complexion seems pale and grey? A bronzer (powder, gel, or cream) instantly conjures up a sun-kissed look. Alternatively, use a CC cream (colour correcting cream) under your foundation. These contain pigments designed to brighten your skin tone. Apricot and pink shades help tired, grey skin appear fresher.

... I have a red nose thanks to constant sniffles?
Concealer in cream form is particularly strongly pigmented and best for covering this type of blemish. At night, apply an ointment containing panthenol or zinc. This facilitates the healing process and reduces any redness.

... I've piled on too many styling products and now my hair looks greasy? If you've just added a bit too much, spray on some dry shampoo, massage it in, and brush out thoroughly. For a real crisis, unfortunately the only solution is washing!

... my lips are chapped? Really simple: dab on honey, let it work for ten minutes, lick it off, and apply some lip balm – this will give you super soft lips.

... the area around my eyes seems really wrinkled?
Dab on a rich eye balm with a high proportion of lipids or an eye cream with hyaluronic acid. Both of these will plump up the skin slightly, thus producing an anti-wrinkle effect.

THE WORST BEAUTY CRIMES

For beauty's sake, avoid these bad habits at all costs:

• Forcibly squeezing spots
• Tearing cuticles
• Excessively plucking eyebrows
• Constantly moistening lips with your tongue (this dries them out)
• Too frequent face scrubs and peels
• Constant frowning
• Consuming too much sugar and alcohol
• Frequently propping your chin on your hand (spot alert!)

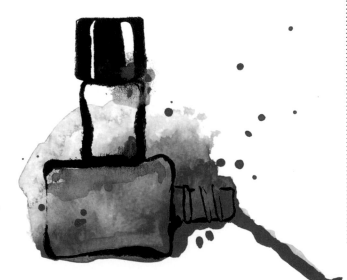

Elegance
from Head
to Toe

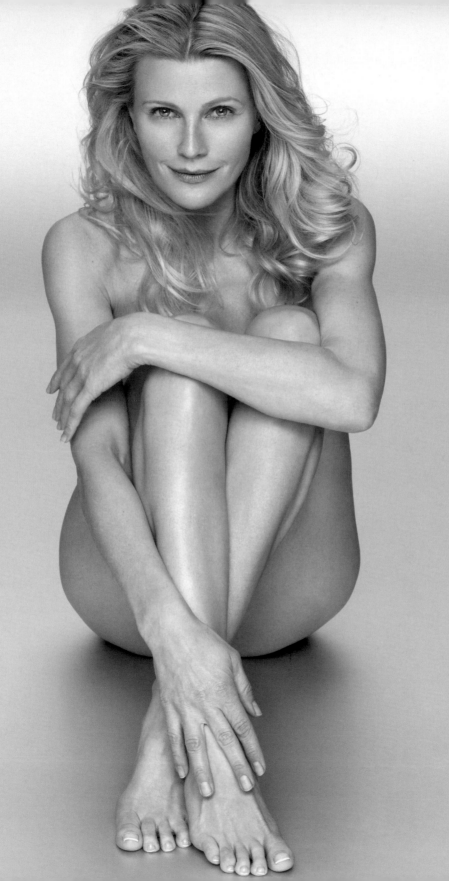

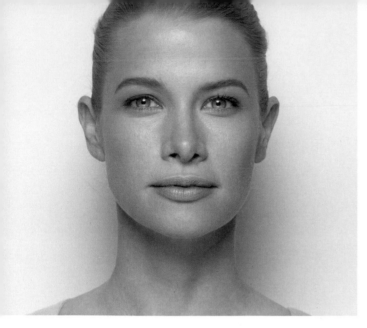

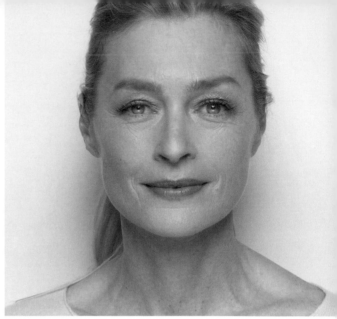

How skin changes

Our skin ages as we do. It is worth knowing how to gently but effectively combat this process.

40+ Wake up tired skin cells

Along with the first small wrinkles caused by dry skin, some expression lines are forming. The lines around the nose and mouth (known as the nasolabial folds) are also becoming deeper. From the age of 40, cell division becomes more sluggish and blood flow through the skin reduces, diminishing the supply of oxygen and nutrients to the cells. As a consequence, dead skin cells remain on the surface for longer, giving the complexion a slightly grey and sallow appearance. Smokers in particular will be likely to notice this.

During this decade you should prioritize repair and protection. The ideal products for this are foundations and moisturizing creams containing antioxidants, which act as cell protectors, as well as light-protection filters to protect against skin damage from UV radiation. The active ingredient vitamin A (retinol) is a powerful weapon in this respect. It stimulates the formation of new collagen fibres in the connective tissue and revitalizes sluggish skin cells.

50+ Soothe red cheeks

As the menopause begins, our skin continues to change. The production of the hormones oestrogen and progesterone decreases, making the skin drier and more sensitive. There is a reduction in collagen and elastin fibres in the connective tissue, which causes the chin, eyelids, and cheeks to sag slightly, and facial contours become increasingly indistinct. In addition, the skin's blood vessels are often weakened and enlarged. This is known as couperose. Fine bluish-red veins are revealed, particularly on the cheeks and at the nostrils, and these become distinctly more visible with stress, heat, spicy food, vigorous exercise, or a glass of wine. Couperose can be a precursor to the skin ailment rosacea, which is associated with an almost permanent reddening of the

Two to three litres of water per day can help the skin appear visibly firmer.

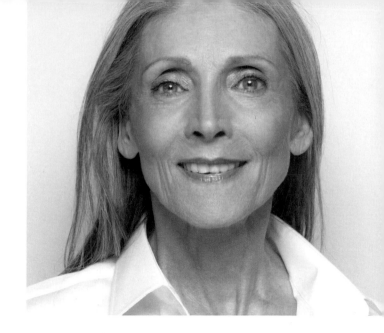

face, often with small pustules similar to acne on the cheeks and around the nose.

It is important to use skincare products with active ingredients that promote the exchange of substances between the cells in the various skin layers, leading to improved collagen production. Special creams that increase vascular strength can help combat couperose. With rosacea, it's vital to avoid oily skincare products. Where there is significant redness or extensive affected areas, you should consult a dermatologist, who can prescribe treatment for the condition.

60+ Repair sun damage

By this age, oestrogen levels have reached their lowest point. The skin is usually very dry and also thinner and more sensitive. This can trigger redness, irritation, an unpleasant taut sensation, itchiness, and sometimes even eczema, which is exacerbated by skin dryness.

In addition, pigment production is often impaired due to too much previous sun exposure. This leads to an increase in melanin production. The visible consequences are brownish-grey pigmentation marks on the face, throat, and backs of the hands. These are also known as age spots or liver spots. Special preparations, referred to as whitening creams, can very

gradually dispel this unwanted pigmentation, or at least lighten it. Particularly troublesome spots can be removed by a dermatologist (see p.150). As a preventative measure, sun protection is strongly recommended. Your daily moisturizer, foundation, and hand cream should have an SPF of at least 15.

70+ Fighting gravity

In this decade it isn't wrinkles and lines that bother us most, but the loss of elasticity in the skin. Sagging skin is particularly noticeable in the cheek areas and at the chin. The skin cells' ability to regenerate has reduced significantly, and in many places the skin is almost parchment thin and transparent, very sensitive, and dry. This is particularly apparent around the eyes: the already thin skin in this area seems even more transparent, with shadows and bags under the eyes appearing to be inevitable.

Daily skincare routines should be as multifunctional as possible. The skin requires high moisture levels and also nourishing lipids and other ingredients that provide a firming and regenerative impact. The perfect solution is provided by creams and foundations containing light-reflecting pigments that have a soft focus effect on the complexion.

Everyday care

Don't use a scatter-gun approach to your skincare; be targeted and specific. In order to achieve the best possible results, take note of your skin type when choosing your skin product's ingredients and consistency.

Simply serene: normal skin

Normal skin is relatively rare. It's fairly uncomplicated, but still needs a bit of attention. Cleansing should be as gentle as possible. Ideally, use a refreshing cleansing gel with relatively low levels of surfactants (you can tell this by the fact that they don't lather particularly strongly). In hard-water areas, an alcohol-free facial toner is ideal for post cleansing; this will remove any last traces of calcium or cleanser from the skin. The ideal skincare cream is one with a high moisture content and which also contains lipids, because over the age of 40, the skin isn't able to produce these in the same quantities as before. A good eye cream is indispensable. For normal skin, a moisturizing product with hyaluronic acid or urea is sufficient.

A delicate flower: sensitive skin

With increasing age, the skin becomes more sensitive. This is caused by a more permeable barrier layer. Sensitive skin reacts quickly to external influences. Wind, heat, and cold can be just as irritating as the wrong kind of skincare product. Even pure water can sometimes be responsible for creating red patches of skin.

For cleansing, use a very mild cleansing lotion or cream without any fragrance or colourings. Micellar lotions, which can be used without water, are also great. They are simply removed with a cotton wool pad or tissue. Afterwards apply a skin cream containing

> Feel free to occasionally veer away from your usual skincare routine; the changing seasons and hormonal skin fluctuations make different demands.

soothing substances that restore the skin's barrier layer, such as algae and liquorice extract, bisabolol or allantoin. Any occasional sensitive spots can be treated using soothing thermal water or algae extract. Always use unscented eye cream.

Constantly thirsty: dry skin

After 40, skin is often dry. The reason for this is that it is less capable of storing moisture than in the past, and what's more, the sebaceous glands operate at a reduced tempo. So even with cleansing products, the focus should be on richness. Creamy, moisturizing cleansing lotions or oils with emollient properties are particularly beneficial. Your facial toner should be alcohol-free and subsequent skincare products should contain moisture-binding ingredients such as hyaluronic acid, glycerine, or aloe vera. Also important are skin-friendly lipids, such as plant oils from almonds, avocado, or grape seed, which strengthen the skin's barrier layer.

Perfect complementary treatment: once a week apply a hydrating face mask (fleece masks are particularly effective). Since the area under the eyes is especially dry, your eye cream should be rich and contain plant oils or shea butter. A waxy eye balm is ideal.

Shiny: oily skin

Women with late onset acne frequently continue to suffer from greasy skin even beyond their 40th birthday:

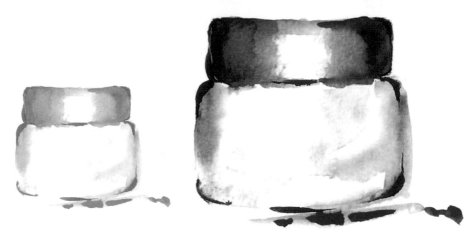

their skin is shiny again just a short time after applying face powder, and make-up is prone to "slipping". Unhelpfully, this is a condition that often persists throughout life.

Mature oily skin must be carefully made less greasy, but it still requires a lot of moisture. For cleansing it is best to use a gentle foam or soap-free lotion; any toner must have a low alcohol content. Skincare products must be specifically geared towards the needs of more mature oily skin. Suitable products may contain zinc, which helps regulate sebum production and has anti-inflammatory properties, and keratolytic (exfoliating) hydroxy acids, along with moisture-enhancing glycerine and wrinkle-reducing substances. A moisturizing eye gel that also reduces puffiness will provide protection against wrinkles.

Undecided: combination skin

Looking after combination skin is a balancing act, thanks to its two completely contrasting needs. Skin in the T-zone (forehead, nose, chin) is usually pretty oily and shiny, while the cheek areas can be extremely dry and have a tendency to develop red patches. For cleansing the entire face, the best product is a soap-free emulsion, as this will not dry out the already dry skin any further. Next, take a cotton pad that has been gently soaked in a low alcohol content facial toner and go over the T-zone. A light, oil-free, highly moisturizing skin cream should also be applied to these areas. Drier areas such as the cheeks will benefit from application of a richer cream containing skin-friendly lipids or even a specific, gentle anti-couperose cream. For the delicate area around the eyes, a light gel cream is perfect.

HOW TO CHECK YOUR SKIN TYPE

In the morning, wash your face with a mild cleansing gel, dab it dry, and then do not moisturize. After 2 or 3 hours, look in the mirror: if your whole face is shiny, you have oily skin. That is pretty rare after the age of 40, but not unheard of. If shiny skin is only evident in the T-zone (forehead, nose, chin), then you have a combination skin type. Does the skin feel really taut? Then you have dry skin. Normal skin can be recognized by the fact that it isn't shiny and feels smooth. Sensitive skin is prone to red patches if not looked after by using protective skincare products.

Protection for the skin

Environmental influences put a severe strain on our skin and can accelerate the ageing process. Skin enemy number one is sunshine – a comprehensive sunscreen is the most effective protection.

The sun makes us look old

A little test: cast an eye over the upper surface of your lower arm. Turn the arm over and look at the underside. This is a good way to see what sunshine does to our skin. While the upper side is slightly tanned, has an uneven skin tone, is more wrinkled and drier, the underside is paler, smoother, and has fewer blemishes – quite simply, it looks much younger.

UV radiation is differentiated into short-wave UVB and long-wave UVA. Both are damaging to your complexion, and even infrared radiation is suspected of facilitating a reduction of collagen in the skin's connective tissue, which in turn leads to a loss of elasticity.

Depending on the location, time of year, and your skin type, it can take a matter of minutes for UVA radiation to trigger an inexorable ageing process. UVA rays penetrate deep into the basal cell layer and inhibit the regeneration of connective tissue cells. This makes the skin thinner, less elastic, and more wrinkled. UVA light also promotes the development of free radicals. These highly reactive oxygen molecules can also attack and modify cell nuclei.

UVB rays likewise trigger inflammatory processes in the skin cells, including damage to your DNA. Minor DNA damage can be repaired by the body, but in the worst cases – if the damage is too great – it can lead to skin cancer.

> A guaranteed tan without damage to your skin or additional wrinkles? Self-tanning lotion or a professional spray tan will conjure up sun-kissed, healthy skin in no time!

Sun protection is wrinkle protection

Good UV protection is the best way to prevent cell damage and premature wrinkles. Many experts advise using products with UV protection on your face all through the year. This doesn't necessarily have to mean using a sun cream. Many tinted moisturizers, foundations, and BB creams have an integrated sun protection factor of between 15 (an often recommended minimum) and 30. In the summer and when on holiday, daily sun protection is essential.

The sun protection factor multiplied by your skin's own self-protection time gives you the length of time you can spend in the sun with a clear conscience. Here's an example: you are fair-skinned and, with no sun protection, you would burn after around five minutes. By using a sun cream with a protection factor of 50, you should safely be able to spend five times 50 minutes (that's about 4 hours) in the sun.

Dermatologists recommend only staying out for around two-thirds of this time before relocating to the shade. Even there you will go brown, admittedly more slowly, but also in a way that is far kinder to your skin than being in the direct sun.

No more excuses!

In the past, applying sun protection was a rather laborious process. The texture was sticky and thick, making it hard to spread, and the whitening effect of

BURNING ISSUES

Most people use too little sun cream, and so don't achieve the protection factor indicated on the packaging. A rule of thumb: to apply sufficient cream from head to toe, you need around 30–40ml (1–1½fl oz). In order to maintain full sun protection, this should be reapplied every 2 hours.

The skin around the eyes is particularly sensitive and it's important to use a special sun cream. These products contain oils that cannot seep into the eyes, are alcohol-free, and usually enriched with anti-ageing ingredients such as hyaluronic acid or vitamin E. A pair of sunglasses will protect you from wrinkles from squinting.

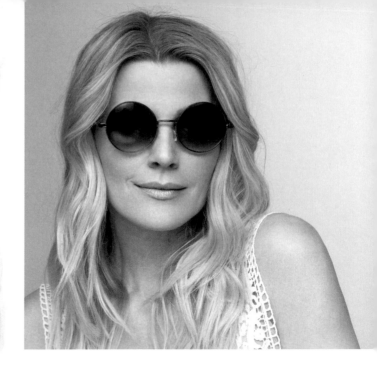

physical light protection filters was not particularly appealing. What's more, the fragrance of lots of these products took some getting used to. But now these drawbacks are things of the past. The latest sunscreen gels and transparent sprays feel really light on the skin, are not oily, and can be applied in a flash. Even suntan oils, which were popular in the 1980s, have undergone a massive improvement. Where their consistency once meant that these products could only achieve a sun protection factor of 4 or 6, now – thanks to special polymers – very high protection factors of 30, 40, or even 50 are attainable.

The industry has tackled the whitening effect of physical barriers such as zinc oxide or titanium dioxide by using ultra-fine ground pigment particles, also called nanoparticles. However, these are not totally uncontroversial – some think they could penetrate the skin if there is any surface damage. For this reason, other companies are focused on a different solution: adding beige-coloured mineral pigments to disguise the whitening effect, which also allows the sun cream to work like a slightly tinted moisturizer, concealing any small skin irregularities. Current products mask the smell of the sun-filtering chemical substances with pleasant fragrances derived from flowers, vanilla, and natural essential oils.

Caught out by the cold

Out of the cold wind and into the dry central heating – the constant temperature fluctuations in winter are particularly challenging for the skin, robbing it of its natural moisture. As a result, skin can become dry, itchy, and scaly. When temperatures outside fall to below just 8 °C (46°F) your sebaceous glands slow down and produce fewer protective oils. Moisturizing creams designed for winter should, therefore, be richer and contain skin-friendly lipids. Water-in-oil emulsions offer long-lasting protection. Pay particular attention to drier areas of your face, such as the delicate lip and eye areas. More luxuriant skincare products that include shea butter, beeswax, or carnauba wax are perfect. The skin on your body, which is often even drier, will benefit from creams that include moisture-promoting substances such as urea, glycerine, or hyaluronic acid, combined with plant oils.

If exposed to extreme cold for longer periods of time, skin should be protected with special barrier creams to avoid damage and to prevent any tendency towards redness from worsening. Thick creams with a high proportion of beeswax or shea butter form a protective coating on the skin against the cold. Take care to wash these off when you get inside, so you don't get a build-up of heat underneath.

It's all in the cleansing

One thing is certain: your skin should be cleansed twice daily, removing any traces of sebum, dirt, and make-up. Lots of cleansers are available – from foaming gels, cleansing oils, and lotions, to exfoliating brushes. Here is a "Who's Who" of cleaning aids for a beautiful complexion.

Cleansing milk

This is a classic cleanser and the perfect partner for normal to dry or sensitive skin. Instead of cleaning the skin using foaming and sometimes aggressive surfactants, cleansing milks contain gentle lipids that lift any dirt, sebum, and make-up from the skin. Depending on the product, the cleanser is applied to dry or slightly damp skin, massaged in using gentle circular motions, and either rinsed off with water or using a cotton wool pad or tissue.

Cleansing gel and foam

Anyone with normal, oily, or combination skin will be well served by a cleansing gel or foam. These cleanse the skin thoroughly with detergent substances such as sodium laureth sulphate, or milder surfactants, such as coconut and maize. If you have sensitive or dry skin but like the fresh sensation of these cleansing products, you should rinse the skin thoroughly with water after use, and perhaps alternate with a richer cleansing product.

Cleansing oil

Oil and water don't go together, right? Wrong. So-called hydrophilic oils are formulated so that the oil is transformed into a refined emulsion when combined with water. This emulsion removes make-up, grease, and dirt from the skin in a particularly gentle manner.

> **Don't overdo it! Too frequent washing removes protective natural lipids and weakens the skin's barrier layer.**

Simply rinse and, thanks to the nourishing effect of the cleansing oil, you often won't even need a moisturizing cream afterwards, at least for normal or combination skin.

Micellar solution

Sometimes sensitive skin won't tolerate any products, and even reacts to water with red patches, raw areas, or a feeling of tightness. The answer is to use a micellar solution; these look like clear water but nonetheless have gentle and effective cleansing properties. They contain both lipophilic (fat-loving) and hydrophilic (water-loving) surfactants. This enables them to envelop any traces of make-up or sebum and to attract dirt particles like a magnet, removing them gently from the skin in one go. Micellar solutions are suitable for removing make-up from the face, but also gentle enough to remove most eye make-up.

Cleansing soap

Normal soaps are strongly alkaline and can dry out and irritate the skin. Special cleansing facial soaps are formulated differently and are available either as a cleansing bar or as a liquid soap. They are adapted to match the skin's pH value, contain mild cleansing substances, and often also emollient oils. Depending on the precise ingredients, they are suitable for dry to oily

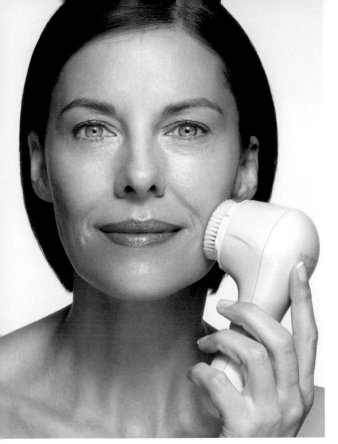

Electronic facial brushes cleanse the complexion particularly thoroughly.

Different types are available for different skin types: those with salicylic acid are good for skin with a tendency to blemishes. If camomile or bisabolol are included in the ingredients, sensitive skin is more likely to tolerate the product.

Exfoliation, brushing, and cleansing sponges

For a proper spring clean you need an exfoliating treatment, a cleansing brush, or facial cleansing sponge (made from the konjac plant or from bamboo fibres). All of these effective tools work in an identical manner: they remove dead flakes of skin, clear the pores, and stimulate circulation. This makes the complexion rosier, more radiant, smoother, and helps avoid the build-up that can cause spots. Oily, normal, or combination skin types can use these products two or three times per week.

Be careful if you have a tendency towards red veins, rosacea, or sensitive skin: physical stimulation of the skin can exacerbate these symptoms. Alternatives include enzyme peel masks, which use a biochemical process to remove dead skin cells, without abrading the skin.

skin types. To use them, create a foam in damp hands, apply in circular movements, and rinse off with plenty of water. Avoid the eye area.

2-in-1 cleanser

Extremely practical if you're short of time in the mornings or get in late at night, these express products combine a cleanser and facial toner. Most are shaken before use and then applied to a cotton wool pad. Wipe this briefly over your face and if necessary repeat with another pad. There is no need to rinse.

Cleansing wipes

Ideal if you're on holiday or you need to remove your make-up quickly before a work-out at the gym, cleansing wipes are impregnated with mild detergent substances and, thanks to their texture, also have a gentle exfoliating effect. Simply run the wipe over your entire face; for heavier make-up use a second or even a third wipe.

CLEANSING THE EYE AREA

For the delicate skin around the eyes, there are various options. If you wear waterproof eye make-up, you'll need a make-up remover containing oil: these usually come in the form of dual-phase solutions. When shaken, you get a homogenous liquid that quickly dissolves make-up without the need for rubbing. A gentle alternative is to use high-quality plant oils, such as almond oil. Non-waterproof mascara, eye shadow, and eyeliner can usually be removed with your regular facial cleansing product. Alternatively, you can use special gentle eye make-up remover lotions, gels, or wipes.

Beauty boosters

Sometimes normal skincare is just not enough. Whatever's bothering you – it might be stress, the drying air at your workplace, or the changing seasons – it's time to call in the elite skincare troops: face masks and serums.

Always a mood enhancer: face masks

Face masks are high-dosage special treatments that can target any skin problems or specific needs more directly than a normal face cream. They also have a more intense impact. This is due to the so-called occlusive effect, which is achieved by applying the mask reasonably thickly. When the air is cut off, warmth builds up and the pores open. This enables nutrients to penetrate the skin more easily and more deeply. Following are some of the most common face mask types and their application.

Anti-ageing/lifting masks are perfect if the skin is showing one too many wrinkles. Anti-ageing masks usually contain a mixture of moisturizing, firming, and nourishing substances, such as hyaluronic acid, and ingredients such as goji berries, or lotus and plant oils. These masks pad out the skin from within; they have a smoothing effect and stimulate collagen production. A similar optical effect is created by lifting masks, which can make the skin seem firmer within a matter of minutes by means of an extremely thin polymer film. **Tip:** always apply to the throat and upper chest too.

Soothing masks help the skin when it becomes irritated due to climatic or seasonal changes, or simply from everyday stress. The soothing mask is laid on like a protective cocoon. It uses skin-friendly lipids from almond, avocado, or macadamia oil to restore the protective barrier that is often damaged in sensitive skin, and it reduces irritation with panthenol, zinc, or thermal water. **Tip:** while using the mask, don't unload the washing machine, just relax on the sofa!

Cleansing masks combat skin impurities that can arise due to stress and hormones. They contain antibacterial ingredients and work rapidly to remove dead skin and refine the pores. They should only ever be applied for a short period of time (between 2 and 5 minutes) or they can have a drying effect, particularly on more mature skin. If there is any tendency towards couperose or rosacea in the cheek areas, just miss these areas out and apply the mask only to the T-zone (forehead, nose, and chin). Finally, cleansing masks, like any other masks, should only be applied to freshly cleansed skin.

Hydrating masks are suitable in the summer or in dry climates, when the skin is crying out for a bit more moisture. Hormonal fluctuations, for example during the menopause, can also result in the skin becoming drier, which makes fine wrinkles more evident. An immediate smoothing effect can be produced by using a hydrating mask containing ingredients such as hyaluronic acid, glycerine, algae, or urea. Not only do these masks supply water to the skin, they also ensure the skin can

> Creamy anti-ageing, lifting, or hydrating masks do not have to be washed off. Gently massage the residue into the skin – this gives you an additional skin-care bonus.

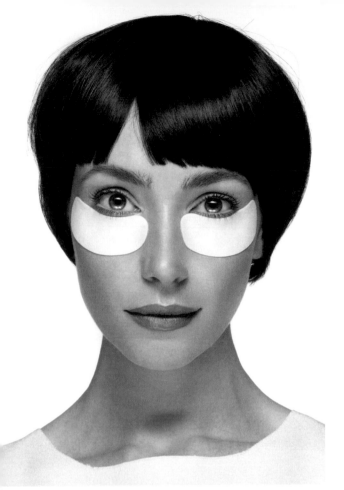

Eye masks enriched with special active ingredients can make circles and puffiness under the eyes disappear in no time. They are cooling and have a plumping effect on the skin.

LIKE A SECOND SKIN ...

There is a special subcategory of masks: hydrating or anti-ageing masks made out of fleece or cellulose, or in the form of silicone gel pads. These masks are laid on the face like a second skin, where they deliver high concentrations of active ingredients. For example, camomile and arnica have a soothing effect on the skin, hyaluronic acid and polysaccharides have intense hydrating properties, and algae extracts and bio-ferments have a powerful firming and smoothing effect.

Fleece and gel masks are not just available for the face as a whole, but there are versions specially shaped for the eye and neck areas. All are applied to clean skin for 10 to 15 minutes. Once removed, there's no need to rinse with water or to apply cream.

retain the moisture better. **Tip:** unlike some masks, hydrating masks can also be applied to the delicate area around the eyes.

Peel-off masks are a classic, in part because they are such fun to use. Peel-off masks are usually transparent; they are applied in a thin layer onto the face and they dry relatively quickly to form a strong film. After the specified treatment time, this film is pulled away from the face, working from the chin upwards. Peel-off masks have a refining impact on the pores and make the skin firmer and less shiny. **Tip:** do not use peel-off masks on very sensitive or dry skin, and take care to avoid the delicate eye area.

Total concentration: serums and ampoules
Serums and ampoules have certain crucial benefits over normal skin creams: they are highly concentrated and therefore have a rapid, more immediately visible effect on the skin. Concentrated ingredients are perfect for targeting specific skin problems. Whether the skin appears creased, washed-out, or stressed, ampoules and serums can make it look better, fresher, and smoother after just a single use.

These beauty boosters can be used as a regular treatment or just when the skin needs urgent help. The concentrated ingredients come in the form of gels or creams, as a spray, as capsules, or ampoules. Particularly potent are the one-use ampoules that contain no preservatives. These contain the precise quantity for a single application and are only opened just before use.

Radiant
in three steps

1 Exfoliation acts as a wake-up call for Almuth's tired complexion. It stimulates the circulation and facilitates absorption of the active substances to follow. The skin looks rosier and more even.

2 Next a face mask pampers the skin. After 10 to 15 minutes the effects are clearly visible: the complexion is smoother and firmer, and little wrinkles appear to have been ironed out.

3 A transparent serum fluid is then massaged into the skin using small circular movements, and is gently patted in under the eyes. This stimulates the lymph circulation, reduces any puffiness, and makes for a truly radiant complexion.

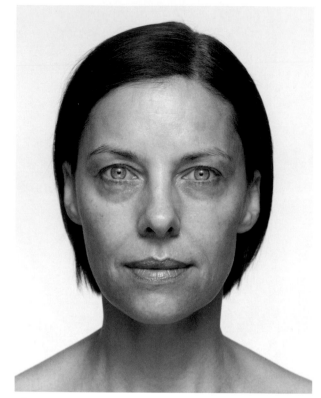

1

Make your own masks

CLAY MASK TO COMBAT REDNESS

Ingredients:
3 tbsp white kaolin clay
3 tbsp mallow tea
3 tbsp rose tea
1 drop each of camomile and lavender essential oils

How it's done: Mix together all the ingredients and apply in a thick layer to the face. Leave to work for 20 minutes. Soften with a lukewarm compress (a damp flannel) and rinse off with plenty of lukewarm water. Moisturize the skin thoroughly afterwards.

GRAPE SEED OIL COMPRESS FOR TIRED SKIN

Ingredients:
1 tbsp grape seed oil
2 tbsp natural yogurt

How it's done: Stir the oil into the yogurt and apply the mask to the face, throat, and neckline. Leave to work for 15 minutes and rinse off with lukewarm water.

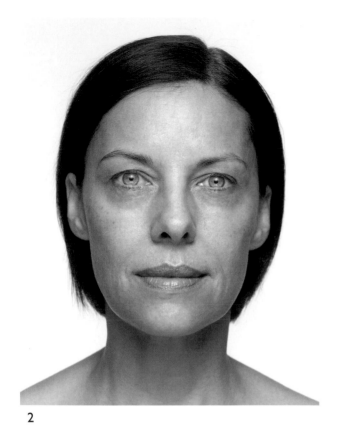

2

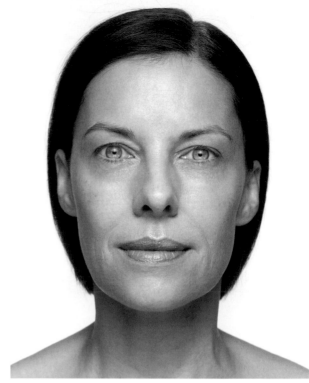

3

AVOCADO MASK TO COMBAT DRYNESS

Ingredients:
½ ripe avocado
2 tbsp whipping cream
1 tsp lemon juice

How it's done: Remove the avocado flesh from the skin and mash with a fork. Stir the cream and lemon juice into the pulp. Apply the mask and leave to work for 15 minutes. Rinse off with warm water. Further skincare is not usually needed afterwards, thanks to the high fat content of the avocado and cream.

FIRMING EGG WHITE MASK FOR THE EYE AREA

Ingredients:
1 egg white
2 tsp coffee grounds
1 tsp evening primrose oil

How it's done: Stir all the ingredients together, put a small quantity onto half a cotton wool pad, and press on under the eyes. Leave to work for 15 to 20 minutes, remove the cotton pad, and rinse with clear water. Finally, apply an eye-care product.

"I am so grateful to my body"

Martina has worked as a model for over 30 years. Her recipe for success involves discipline and taking good care of herself. Anything she demands from her body, she tries to repay twofold.

I t's almost enough you make you envious: at this photo shoot Martina is "permitted" to loll about in a warm bath full of colourful rose petals. But in the enormous loft apartment where this morning's shooting is taking place, it is cold enough to make your teeth chatter. While superficially it appears fun, it is clear to everyone that this is hard work. Denise, the photographer, readjusts the lighting over and over again, and relentlessly requests changes to posture and pose. This continues until, after three-quarters of an hour, she is finally happy with the results. By this point the bath water is only lukewarm, but Martina is still smiling. Ever the professional.

"I've always known that this job could be over at any time"

Without a doubt, this 49-year-old understands all the ins and outs of her job. Martina has been modelling for over 30 years; she was approached by an agency scout on the streets of Cologne at the age of 16. She still remembers her first photographs. They were for a men's jeans catalogue. "My role was as a kind of American girl accessory for the male models. The image of women was rather different in those days … "

She entered a competition for the magazine *Carina* and won first prize – a contract with a Munich model agency. Her first foreign jobs soon followed.

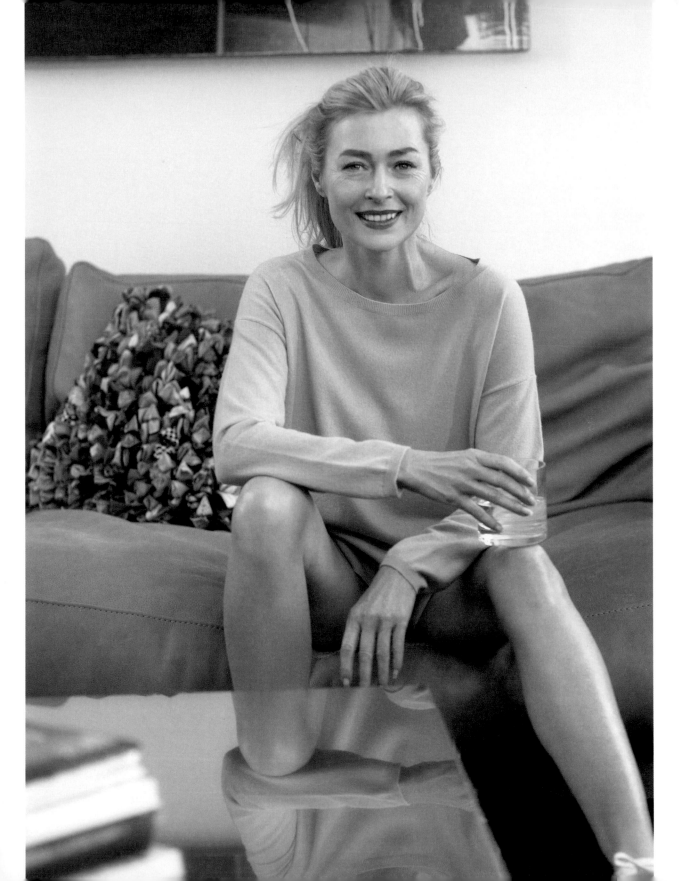

Martina loves the whirlwind lifestyle of a model and the constant back and forth between big cities, but she didn't lose focus and went on to complete her schooling. "My parents insisted on it. They were incredibly proud of me, but they also knew that a job reliant on beauty can have a very short shelf life," explains Martina. Once she was 18 and had successfully completed her studies, she began full-time work as a model. Soon she was up in front of the camera for fashion companies all over the world: one day a beauty shoot in a spa in Mexico, the next day sporty outfits in Australia. "In those days there was a lot more money in the industry for advertising than there is today. I really made it, the classic dream job for so many young girls," she says.

"After the birth of my son, my perspective on things changed"

At 28 Martina became pregnant with a longed-for child. For 3 years she didn't work, but was able to live off the proceeds of the preceding years. "I didn't then know whether I would be able to make a fresh start in the modelling business once I was over 30," she remembers. But it was important to her to spend the first years of her son's life very close to him. "It always sounds like such a cliché and rather cheesy, but that time is irreplaceable and it gave me a whole new perspective on the world," says Martina.

In fact, she was lucky: the industry was just beginning to pay attention to models who were 30 and 40+. Anti-wrinkle creams could now finally be advertised by their actual target group. Martina successfully restarted her career after her 3-year break. And when she was away travelling for longer periods for a shoot somewhere in the world, her own mother looked after her son. "But this balancing act wasn't always so simple. Particularly if a well-paid job came along at short notice, meaning I then had to organize everything in a real rush." Things were no different for her than for many other women who juggle jobs and children. "My mother was such a great support during this time and I knew that my son was getting the best care from her. Even so, I sometimes felt guilty," she remembers.

"If I had been unhappy, I wouldn't have looked beautiful either"

This 49-year-old might have an abundance of good genes, but Martina doesn't take it for granted. "I feel so grateful for my body. And over the years I've learned that anything I demand from it, I must repay in kind at least twice over."

When she has free time, she loves to run with her dog through woods and parks. Three times a week she does some strength training at the gym. She doesn't smoke or drink alcohol; she eats very little meat, but consumes plenty of fruit, vegetables, and dairy products. If she is in a rush or needs a little snack while on a job, her favourite thing is a smoothie: "You can mix one up in no time, it's really filling, and I know it's super healthy for me too." The days of going out partying after work are long since over. Today she goes to bed early and needs lots of sleep. "That might sound like typical beauty advice from a model, but I do it primarily for myself. And I feel really great with this lifestyle," she explains. She is in a relationship that makes her happy. "Body, mind, and soul have to be in harmony. If I was unhappy, I wouldn't look beautiful." She accepts that she has lines around the eyes and mouth, just like any other woman of her age, and it doesn't annoy her in the slightest. "I've lived a bit and I don't want to be lying in a coffin at the age of 80 looking in immaculate condition." She would never consider cosmetic surgery. But "I respect women who do make that choice." When she does find a bit of time for herself in her limited free hours, she loves to read. Right now she is reading books on mindfulness.

Martina's favourite smoothie

This fruity orange and raspberry smoothie is simultaneously delicious and healthy – it contains an abundance of vitamin C and antioxidants.

For 2 glasses:
250g (9oz) raspberries (ideally organic)
250ml (9fl oz) orange juice (organic, if possible)
200g (7oz) natural yogurt (3.5% fat)
honey to taste
mint leaves to garnish

Preparation:
Purée all the ingredients in a blender, pour into two glasses, and decorate with mint leaves.

Anti-ageing ingredients

New products are constantly being marketed that supposedly make the skin look younger, firmer, and smoother. But which ones really do counteract the effects of ageing? Here are the rejuvenating ingredients currently recommended by dermatologists.

Antioxidants

Antioxidants are contained in many skincare products. They comprise a whole range of substances with a single common objective: combating free radicals. Free radicals are highly reactive oxygen molecules that attack our skin cells, making us age visibly. They multiply under the impact of sunlight or environmental factors, but are also produced by the body itself.

Antioxidants include vitamins C and E, beta-carotene, green tea extracts, resveratrol from grapes, and also trace elements such as selenium, copper, and zinc. These neutralize free radicals, making them harmless.

Ascorbic acid (vitamin C)

This water-soluble vitamin acts as a protective shield for the skin cells. It intercepts free radicals that try to attack the cell nucleus. In addition, it helps the skin produce more collagen, thus keeping the connective tissues firm. If vitamin C combines with vitamin E, it can enhance the latter's cell-protecting effect. Since vitamin C is not produced by the body itself, we must consume it as part of our diet. This miracle vitamin is also included as an active ingredient in some skincare products.

Ceramides

These molecules include the natural dermatological lipids that act as building blocks in the fat in the outermost layer of the epidermis. They protect the skin against dehydration and make it smooth and more resistant to external environmental influences. With increasing age, the quantity of ceramides in the skin falls. Skincare products therefore often incorporate plant ceramides to compensate for this loss.

Coenzyme Q10

Q10 assists the little power generators in our cells, the so-called mitochondria, in producing energy. In addition, this coenzyme neutralizes free radicals and can protect skin against sun and environmental damage, as well as from premature wrinkles. To a certain extent the body

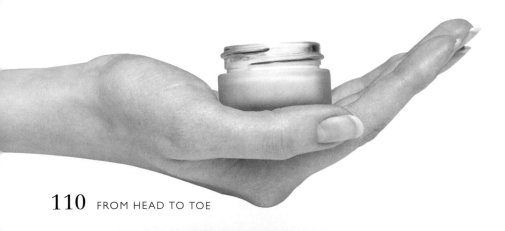

can produce Q10 itself, but over the course of time these deposits diminish, because Q10 production gets put on the back burner from around your mid-30s.

Since this coenzyme also strengthens the immune system, heart and nerves, you should seek it out in both your skincare products and your diet. Meat, fish, nuts, and broccoli contain particularly high quantities of Q10.

Elastin

This is a protein that forms the main component of the flexible fibres in our connective tissue. With increasing age, these fibres become thoroughly worn out and stretched. The consequence: skin is less firm and becomes wrinkled. High-tech processes can be used to incorporate animal elastin into skin creams, to encourage younger, more flexible fibres in the connective tissue.

Yeast

Some forms of yeast produce highly effective antioxidants and strengthen the skin's barrier layer by boosting the body's natural lipid production. In addition, it can send signals to the deeper skin layers, so that more collagen fibres are produced. The result is that the skin is more padded from within and minor wrinkles are smoothed out. The cell walls in yeast contain sugar compounds (beta-glucans) that are thought to strengthen the skin's immune cells. Skincare products containing yeast are ideal for those with sensitive skin or allergies.

THE FUTURE FOR SKIN

There is a lot going on in the laboratories of big cosmetic companies. For example, scientists are researching the possibility of individually adapting cosmetics depending on someone's genetic make-up. From the results of one blood test, an individually formulated cream could provide your skin with precisely the additional support that nature has deprived it of. There is still a long way to go before that can be achieved, though.

But it may not be long at all before beauty products come onto the market that are designed to function with the skin's biorhythms, releasing specific active ingredients at particular times, depending on what the skin needs most urgently at different points in the day. For example, degreasing substances could be activated around midday, when the sebaceous glands are at their most active.

Hyaluronic acid

A much-praised, commonly used ingredient – and quite rightly. Nowadays this skin-flattering substance is usually produced synthetically. It acts like a little sponge, holding an enormous quantity of water in the skin, leaving it looking firm, radiant, and youthful. Scientists are currently researching how they might get this super-ingredient to penetrate into the deeper skin layers: one approach is to use microcapsules of hyaluronic acid; another is to fractionate the substance, breaking it down into little pieces that can penetrate the skin more easily than larger molecules.

The right cream can work miracles.
Skin that has been well looked after
over the years will still look vibrant,
fresh, and radiant in later life, even
with a few wrinkles.

Hydroxy acids

Powerful allies in the fight against wrinkles are alpha, beta, and poly hydroxy acids (AHA, BHA, PHA), also known as fruit acids. They occur naturally in apples, grapes, sugar cane, and milk. When used in skincare, they are often reproduced in a laboratory. They remove old flaky skin cells, have an intensive exfoliating effect, and leave the skin with finer pores, smoother, softer, and as radiant as if it has been freshly polished.

Hydroxy acids occur in low concentrations in cleansing products, facial toners, and in creams; and in higher concentrations in the chemical peels used by dermatologists and beauticians. Beta and poly hydroxy acids are more suitable for sensitive skin, since they are considerably gentler than alpha hydroxy acids.

Peptides

Recently peptides have become star performers in the beauty sector. Consisting of protein chains made of two or more amino acids, they are used in cosmetic products in the form of polypeptides, oligopeptides, tripeptides, and dipeptides. They get sluggish cell regeneration up and running again, and ensure that the interaction between the different individual skin layers functions more effectively. This has the effect of making more mature skin behave as though it was much younger, with the result that it appears firmer and more radiant.

Phytohormones

These rejuvenating hormones are of particular interest for women experiencing the menopause, whose natural hormone production is reduced, resulting in imbalances in the body. These cause the skin to become thinner, drier, and more sensitive, as well as losing the padding of subcutaneous fat tissues. Phytohormones are derived from soya, shiitake mushrooms, hops, and also from the South American yam root. They have an effect similar to that of oestrogen, but without the potential side effects caused by "real" hormones. They help the skin to store more moisture and aid in the creation of more collagen and elastin – resulting in a firmer, smoother appearance.

Retinol (vitamin A) and vitamin A acid

For decades dermatologists have recognized retinol as an effective weapon against wrinkles. This highly potent substance works on multiple levels: it boosts the production of new skin cells, stimulates formation of fibres in the connective tissue, repairs skin damage, aids the development of new supply channels to the cells, and even contributes moisture. However, it can irritate sensitive skin, and makes skin more sensitive to the effects of sunlight. The amounts allowed in over-the-counter skincare products are therefore strictly limited.

Vitamin A acid is a much stronger derivative of vitamin A and only available in prescription products. It is primarily used in the form of creams or tablets for treating acne, but it is also an effective anti-wrinkle agent, even in very low doses.

Oxygen

Cells must be supplied with sufficient oxygen if the skin is to look radiant, smooth, and healthy. Unfortunately, our cells' oxygen content has already begun to diminish by around the age of 25. Stress and smoking both reduce the proportion of oxygen in the cells even more dramatically. The quickest way to top up oxygen deposits is to take a deep breath, ideally when outside in the fresh air and while moving briskly. But face creams and serums are also available that have been enriched with this powerful substance.

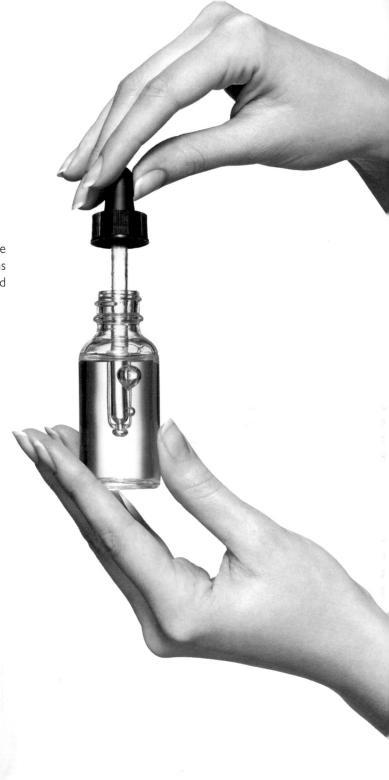

VEGETABLE DYES AS A FOUNTAIN OF YOUTH

In the USA, everyone is talking about senolytics or senolytic substances being the great anti-ageing success story. The main representative of this group of substances is the yellow vegetable dye quercetin, which can be found in apples, broccoli, green beans, and grapes, among other things. It eliminates old cells in the body that (similarly to cancer cells) are resistant to programmed cell death (apoptose), and by doing so it can considerably slow down the ageing process. Quercetin is available in capsules, but is also increasingly included as an ingredient in face creams.

A radiant smile

Even teeth cannot escape the ageing process. They look more transparent, edges become more brittle, and discolouration can occur. Correct care and professional treatments can combat these effects.

A matter of cleanliness

The groundwork is daily dental care at home. Whether you prefer a standard toothbrush or an electric brush is up to you. Electric toothbrushes are a little more gentle on the gums and clean particularly thoroughly thanks to their 48,000 rotations per minute (manual toothbrushes are only around 600 per minute). The crucial thing in both cases is getting the technique right: position the toothbrush at the junction between the tooth and the gum and for each tooth in turn, clean with a gentle back and forth movement from the red (gum) to white (tooth). If you have an electric toothbrush, hold it steady on each tooth, as the machine will take control of the back and forth movements. It is also important to clean the interdental spaces, as these can harbour damaging bacteria. The essential tools for everyday use include dental floss, interdental brushes, and (for dental bridges and braces) specialist orthodontic floss with dental floss threaders. Your dentist will show you how to use these properly.

Keep breath fresh with dental chewing gum, a cup of black tea, or an occasional spoonful of unsweetened natural yoghurt

Professional deep clean

You should aim to have your teeth cleaned professionally twice a year. For a deep clean, the hygienist will remove tartar either manually and/or using ultrasound. A salt-water mix (air flow or air polishing) can then be used to eliminate any discolouration. Then, afterwards, the teeth will be polished.

After the age of 40, regular gum checks should be carried out by the dentist and/or hygienist. Plaque can build up between the teeth and gum tissue, leading to halitosis and inflammation. Bleeding gums are a clear sign that there is a gum problem. Depending on the depth of the gingival pockets around the teeth, these can be cleaned with or without local anaesthetic, using ultrasound and small dental instruments.

Bright and beautiful

You may not want the gleaming blue-white teeth sported by Hollywood stars, but this doesn't necessarily mean putting up with discolouration, which can have an ageing effect. A whitening or brightening toothpaste can make the teeth a touch brighter, but for a more dramatic effect, bleaching with hydrogen peroxide is the answer. It's most effective if carried out by the dentist. Hydrogen peroxide gel in varying concentrations is applied to the teeth and activated using a special light. This produces oxygen that results in the teeth becoming up to nine shades lighter.

It is also possible to whiten your teeth at home using a weaker hydrogen peroxide formula. To do this, your dentist creates a special dental tray that you then fill at home with a bleaching gel and wear for a number of hours over a period of two to three weeks. Depending on your dietary habits (tea, coffee, fruit, and red wine are the main culprits), the results can last for two to three years.

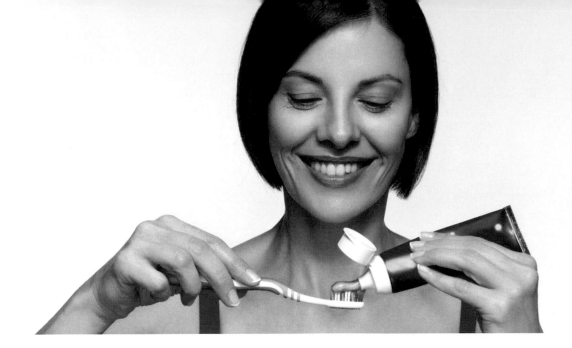

In good shape

Over the course of the years, teeth get worn out. The front teeth often become a bit shorter and their edges develop an uneven appearance. This can make the face look older. Ceramic veneers, which are just 0.3 mm thick, could be the solution. These can be used to correct irregularly shaped teeth and also to conceal any small holes. The veneers are manufactured individually, modelled on a dental impression, and then adhered to the actual tooth. With some techniques, the tooth has to be lightly sanded first. Other so-called "no-prep" veneers can be applied without any loss to the existing tooth. Now the bad news: veneers are extremely expensive. A more affordable option is to opt for composite synthetic veneers, which are moulded layer by layer on the tooth.

Stronghold

The main cause of tooth loss after the age of 40 is periodontitis, a severe type of gum disease that often occurs in those little gaps between the teeth that look like black triangles. Apart from regular preventative interventions, there are treatment options available that can help restore the gums.

BLUE HUES TO COMBAT YELLOWING

Little optical tricks can also be used to make your teeth look whiter. Warm lipstick colours with yellowy undertones, such as red-orange or terracotta colours, make the teeth look yellower, whereas cool tones with hints of blue, such as pink or subtle berry shades, make them appear whiter and brighter.

Even your choice of earrings can have an impact on your teeth! Silver, white gold, or platinum (i.e. cool tones) make the teeth seem brighter. Yellow or rose gold will emphasize any possible yellow shades. Clear gemstones also complement the teeth beautifully, ideally those with a hint of blue, such as aquamarine, beryl, blue sapphires, diamonds, and quartz.

Neck & décolletage

Facial care shouldn't stop at the chin. A firm, smooth neck and upper chest are desirable, but these areas are often neglected when it comes to skincare. This doesn't have to be the case.

Not to be forgotten …

Unfortunately, the throat and upper chest area are naturally rather poorly endowed with the sebaceous glands that ensure smooth and supple skin. In addition, the skin in these areas is very thin and has little subcutaneous fat tissue. This combination results in dry skin that wrinkles easily and has a propensity to lose its elasticity. Specialized throat and bust creams are available to help ensure the skin is well toned and smooth. Along with moisturizing and smoothing substances, these creams also contain tightening ingredients such as peptides or silicone. Alternatively, you can just apply your normal skincare product to the area.

The chest as a barometer of stress

Hot flushes, perspiration, and stress are often particularly noticeable in a woman's neck and chest area. The sensitive skin here reddens easily and random blotches can appear. If this applies to you, use a cream that is specifically formulated for sensitive skin to care for the throat and chest areas, one that contains soothing ingredients, such as shiso or liquorice extract, algae, or thermal plankton. If you need a quick fix, for example before a meeting, a thermal water spray can help eliminate any red blotches. Another good solution is to hold a cold water bottle onto the affected area. In the longer term, learning relaxation methods, such as yoga, or

> Rapid response: special infused silicone pads worn during the day for a few hours will make the upper chest area look truly breath-taking with your low-neck evening wear.

breathing practice, may help calm you and lessen reactions in certain situations. One last tip is to keep a lightweight silk or cotton shawl stashed in your bag. You can use this to conceal any possible hot flushes.

Special protection

The throat and upper chest belong to the body's so-called "sun terraces". This means that UV rays fall almost vertically onto these areas throughout the year, albeit with varying intensity. And since the sun is skin enemy number one, its effects become clearly noticeable over time: along with wrinkles caused by exposure to UV light, pigmentation spots can easily develop in these areas. If these brown-grey persistent discolourations are already present, the only remedy is a lightening cream of some kind. A dermatologist can remove the blotches with a laser. Even better is to avoid them in the first place: use a moisturizing cream in these areas all year round containing a sun protection factor of at least 20, and in summer use a sun cream with SPF 50+.

Anti-wrinkle aids

Along with the right cream, there are a whole host of skincare rituals that will help prevent the development of wrinkles on the throat and around the neckline. Some of these literally work in your sleep. By using a flat, not too soft pillow, and adopting a sleeping position on your back, you will prevent neckline wrinkles in particular. Soft, cuddly pillows, and sleeping on your side or stomach seem to magically attract wrinkles. There are special nighttime bras and sleepwear that hold the breasts more or less in position, and so protect the décolletage area from wrinkling. It does appear to work – but whether or not you can or want to sleep wearing one is something you'll have to discover for yourself.

A small, often underestimated secret weapon is a daily percussion massage, which you can perform when applying your moisturizer. Here's how it's done: spread your day cream or specialized skincare cream over the neck and décolleté areas. Then turn your head to one side and tap in the cream on one side with the flat of your hand, working upwards, before switching sides. Hold the head up straight again and likewise gently tap in the cream from the centre of your lower neckline up towards the chin.

Facial gym for firm contours

Admittedly facial gymnastics look rather idiotic, but they are extremely effective. Like every other muscle in the body, the facial musculature can be trained and toned. No one has to watch you doing it! Position yourself in front of a mirror, wearing no clothes on your upper body. Smile as broadly as possible and say "X". Tense the neck muscles while you are doing this. Then relax the mouth and neck areas again before tensing, smiling, and saying "X" once again. Repeat ten times.

The following exercise tones the neck area: stand up straight, looking forwards. Push your chin forwards and stretch the lower lip over your upper lip. Resist turning the corners of your mouth upwards when doing this. Increase the resistance while pressing gently upwards against the chin with your fist. Press the tongue against the upper incisors. You should be able to detect this movement in the fist under your chin. Hold the tension for five seconds, release gradually, and then repeat the exercise five times.

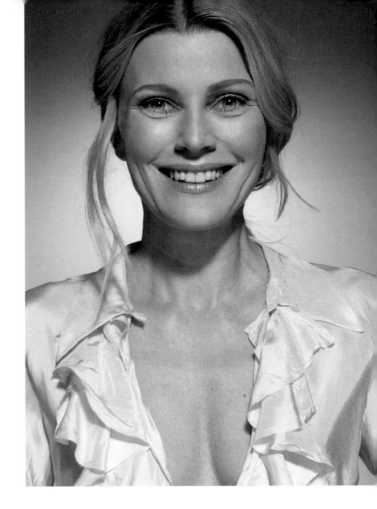

CHEATING IS ALLOWED

For an even more beautiful neckline, feel free to cheat a bit. Red patches can be concealed using a mineral powder foundation, BB cream, or a light liquid foundation. If applied very thinly, these can look completely natural. To give the impression of a deeper cleavage, apply some bronzing powder between the breasts. A shimmering (not glittery) powder or an iridescent oil will have a wonderfully smoothing effect on any little wrinkles.

Care for the body

The skin on your body is usually drier than on the face and neck, and needs special care in order to remain smooth, firm, and supple. Use this as motivation to create a daily skincare ritual and a proper pampering programme.

No need for a flood of foam

Of course, your daily shower should be refreshing and cleansing. But don't overdo it on the foam front. The less a shower gel foams, the gentler it will be. Mild surfactants from coconut and maize will have a far less drying impact on your skin.

If the skin on your body is very dry, shower oils may be the best choice. When these come into contact with water they transform into a milky emulsion, which is easy to rinse off but leaves behind a soothing emollient film on the skin.

So-called in-shower treatments are practical and time-saving. These are applied over the whole body after washing, left to work briefly, and then rinsed off. They work like a kind of body lotion, so using a moisturizer afterwards becomes unnecessary. They don't leave a sticky film behind on the skin and don't need to be absorbed, so you can get dressed straight away afterwards.

Shower and bath products made with natural essential oils may be less likely to irritate the skin than those containing a cocktail of artificial fragrances. But some natural ingredients are irritants, and the body can develop allergies to natural ingredients as well as those from a laboratory. If you have very sensitive skin you should select fragrance-free shower and bath products.

> Stressbuster: direct a firm jet of water from the shower onto the nape of your neck with the temperature as hot as you can tolerate for 3 minutes – the stimulation of the surrounding nerves and nerve cell clusters will relax you instantaneously.

Deep clean the pores of your skin

In some areas of the body (shins, knees, elbows), the skin is naturally endowed with hardly any sebaceous glands, with the consequence that rough skin can easily develop in these areas. Dead skin cells give the skin a grey appearance and chapped or cracked areas are unsightly and can be sore.

To ensure the skin looks healthy and is soft to the touch, use exfoliating treatments in conjunction with massage brushes, gloves, and sponges. Exfoliating body scrubs contain quite coarse abrasive particles made from ground fruit stones or loofah sponge pieces. They are gently massaged into the skin using circular movements and then rinsed off under the shower with lukewarm water. Additional skin care can be provided by sea salt and oil scrub treatments, which leave a slight lipid film on the skin after showering.

When using massage brushes, sponges, or exfoliation gloves, always move in a circular direction on damp skin over the entire body. Body scrubs should not be used more than twice a week, whereas massage sponges and brushes can be used on a daily basis.

Those with sensitive skin should choose exfoliants without abrasive particles: shower gels with mild fruit acids also work to remove dry, dead skin cells.

FROM ORANGE TO PEACH

Cellulite is primarily a problem for women. Connective body tissue is constructed differently in women; it is less strong and thus more malleable than it is in men, something that is advantageous in pregnancy. The connective tissue fibres, which run primarily in parallel, can be more easily penetrated by fat cells, and this results in the typical skin appearance associated with cellulite. A combination of aerobic and strength training can reduce the fat and build muscles, declaring war on that orange-peel skin. Also helpful are lymphatic drainage, daily brush massages, and alternating hot/cold showers. Not a lot of people know that a low-carb diet (less than 50g carbohydrates per day) can dramatically improve the skin's appearance.

Oil on our skin

With increasing age, the skin on the body becomes drier, and is also less firm and elastic. So skincare after showering should be multifunctional: skin-friendly vegetable lipids restore missing oils to the skin, emollient and moisture-binding substances combat the shortage of water, and firming ingredients strengthen the weakened connective tissue. Body creams are generally richer than body lotion or milk. So-called "dry oils" are particularly good for the skin. Thanks to a combination of vegetable and silicone oils, they lie lightly on the skin without making it greasy or sticky.

The middle kingdom

Regularly topping the list of female problem areas is the stomach. You can help it remain smooth during your morning bath routine. Special skincare products to enhance tone and flexibility can help, but standard body oil works fine too. Ideally combine your moisturizing routine with a little pinching massage. Here's how it's done: spread some oil over the stomach area, and using the thumbs and index fingers, pull up little rolls of skin, hold briefly, and then release again. The skin should redden slightly as you are doing this, which is a sign of increased circulation. Finally, rub and stroke with the palm of your hand in large clockwise circles over the stomach. For maximum impact, you'll need to do this pinching massage over an extended period, ideally every day.

The causes of regular stomach bloating can include stress or hormonal imbalances. But nutrition is an even more likely culprit. Alongside the usual suspects like cabbage, pulses, onions, and garlic, it is less well known that for many people excess stomach gases can also be caused by dairy products, strong spices, and sugar substitutes (particularly sorbitol and xylitol). Rapid relief can be provided by drinking tea made from aniseed, fennel, and caraway, or performing a little stomach massage using a couple of drops of mint and basil essential oils dissolved in 25ml of almond oil.

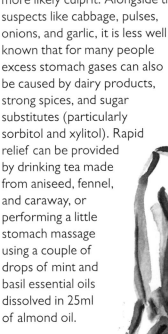

Hair removal

Soft and silky smooth is how we generally prefer our skin to be. Annoying little hairs on the legs, in the armpits, around the bikini area, and on the face are a real inconvenience. This is all you need to know about removing them.

Super-fast: wet shave

The wet shave is the preferred hair removal method for many women. The advantages are obvious: it is quick, painless, and inexpensive. Specially designed razors have gentle, but still very sharp blades. Some versions have integrated skincare strips to ensure that the blade glides more smoothly over the skin and can even be used without shaving foam or gel.

Razors are ideal for removing hair from the legs and armpits. You need to be careful in the bikini area, however. Here you can often get little red spots after shaving. The hairs here are thicker, the follicles larger, and levels of bacteria higher, which is why wet shaving in this area is more likely to lead to inflammation.

It's important to always shave against the hairs' direction of growth, avoid pressing too hard, and don't go over the same spot repeatedly with the razor. The main disadvantage of this method is that the hair grows back quickly, and you may need to re-shave to remove the stubble after just a couple of days.

Twinges slightly: epilation

Epilators pluck out individual hairs at top speed with their rotating tweezers. It doesn't sound like a totally painless procedure, and sadly it isn't. Modern appliances can usually be used dry as well as in the shower or bath. For dry epilation, the skin must be completely free of any grease. Stretch the skin slightly, place the epilator at right angles, and run it gently over the skin, against the direction of hair growth.

Epilation under water is somewhat less unpleasant. Thanks to the warm water, the pores open up and the hairs stand up slightly, which makes the task a bit easier.

Very long hairs should be trimmed before epilation – modern epilators can handle hairs from as short as 0.5mm in length. The main advantage of this method is that the smooth feeling lasts for up to 4 weeks.

Grit your teeth: waxing & sugaring

Should you wax yourself or have it done for you? You can do it yourself, but for a novice it's best to make use of a salon. The staff there are hugely experienced in ways of making the somewhat barbaric process more bearable. But you still can't afford to be too squeamish, because there is no doubt that waxing really hurts, especially the first time. Warm wax is applied to the skin, left briefly to dry – and then is pulled off with a tug against the direction of hair growth. For best results the hairs should be neither too long nor too short – around 5mm is the ideal length.

A less painful alternative, particularly for sensitive skin, is sugaring. This involves a thick paste made from sugar, water, and lemon juice, which is applied while warm to the skin, and then pulled off with kneading movements. Even the finest hairs, from 3mm long, will be caught. The longer the hairs, the more it stings. As a rule, a professional waxing or sugaring procedure will last for between 3 and 6 weeks.

Really simple: depilatory creams

The most unpleasant thing about depilatory creams is the smell of the active ingredient, thioglycolic acid. This dissolves the hair keratin under the surface of the skin, which makes the hairs fall out, and after a few minutes they can be removed with a spatula, or simply showered off along with the cream. The results last for between

4 and 5 days. Sensitive skin can react to these creams, even if they contain soothing additives such as almond oil or shea butter. This is because depilatory creams have a pH value of 12.5, which is much higher than skin's pH of 5.5. So it's important to carry out a tolerance test in the crook of your arm, and to adhere precisely to the prescribed application time.

Lightning quick smoothness: laser epilation

For a number of years now the possibility of hair removal by laser treatment has offered a solution to get rid of hairs on a more permanent basis.

Diode lasers and the closely related flash lamp appliances or IPL (Intensed Pulse Light) equipment use concentrated light with a specific wavelength. The light penetrates the upper skin layers and targets the hair root, which is destroyed so that no hair can regrow in that location. The surrounding tissue is not damaged during the process. The treatment hardly hurts at all, but if necessary an anaesthetic cream can be applied, which will ensure that you feel absolutely nothing. Afterwards, the skin will be slightly reddened and may be a bit swollen too.

Since successful removal of the hairs relies on catching them at a particular phase of growth, between five and seven treatments are required at intervals of 4 to 6 weeks, depending on the precise area of the body. Note that the lighter the skin, the more effective the treatment. Darker and tanned skin cannot be laser treated.

Plucking and threading

While the hair on your head becomes increasingly fine as you grow older, facial hair tends to flourish. Undesirable hairs around the eyebrows and on the upper lip can be removed using slant tweezers and a magnifying mirror. When doing this, only ever pluck out individual hairs rather than whole clusters, and check the results periodically in a standard mirror.

Another option is the oriental hair removal technique of threading, which is carried out by a beautician. This is a super-fast method and is particularly thorough.

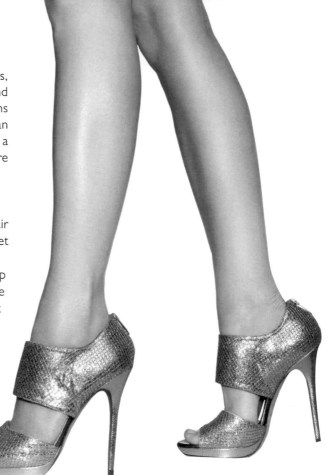

SKIN SOOTHERS

To reduce irritation after epilation, try:
- Baby powder or talcum powder with lavender essential oil
- Pure aloe vera gel, with at least 98% aloe vera content (without added alcohol)
- Placing a gel pack from the fridge on the skin for 5 minutes

"I like to be involved"

Barbara doesn't always find growing older amusing. Her motto is: you stay young if you are interested, on the ball, and speak your mind.

When Barbara arrived at the photo shoot she immediately pounced on a clothes rail and pulled out a full-length, wine-coloured paisley patterned dress. "I had one exactly like this in blue in my student days. That has got to be in the photo."

Before the shooting starts and work gets underway, she is allowed to enjoy herself a bit. In Boris's capable hands the 63-year-old relaxes with eyes closed under a fleece face mask, followed by a little facial massage with a moisturizing serum. Barbara agrees it is blissful, but says "I'm not really the bathroom pampering type. My kind of relaxation involves stimulating conversation and fine food." Or piano playing: "Music is my passion. I've been playing since the age of 8 and can forget all my everyday preoccupations when I'm at the piano." Barbara has only been modelling for eight years, since she was approached one day on the street. Fashion and beauty are not really her area; many of her shoots are for medical or phone companies. After studying textile engineering she worked for various interior design companies. She was previously married and has two sons from that relationship.

"Divorce was liberating for me"

Shortly after her silver wedding anniversary, Barbara decided to separate from her husband. "The separation was instigated by me, but I still wasn't proud of doing it. After such a long time together, it inevitably feels like something

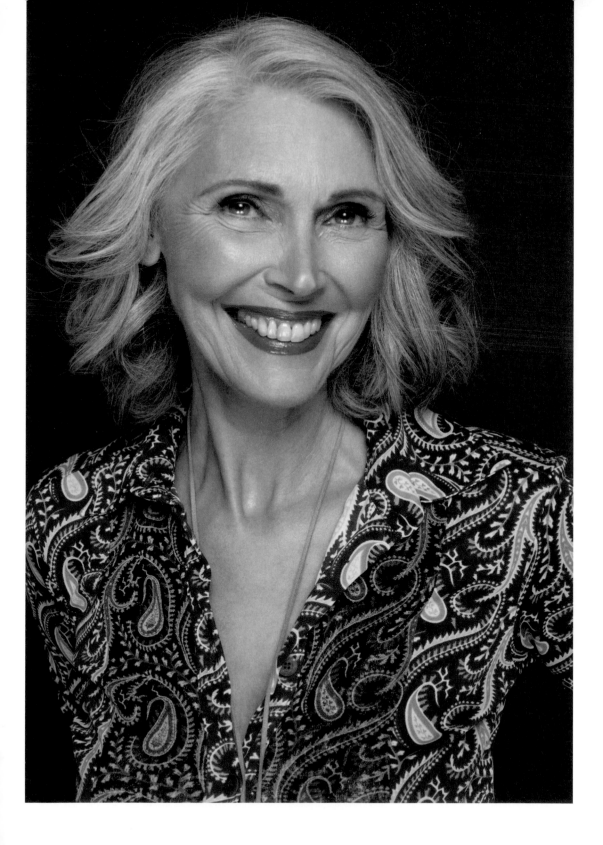

of a defeat. And the question remains, why didn't it work for us when so many other couples manage to stay together?" Nevertheless, she feels the separation was a kind of liberation, and also a brave step towards a fresh start: "It was a gradual process of increasing unease up to a point which is hard to clearly define, until I finally found the courage to take this enormous step with all its consequences." She found it particularly hard that the separation led to the loss of many social connections. "Your friendship circle and acquaintances really divide. Either they remained steadfastly loyal to me, or they sided with my husband."

Meanwhile, she has a new partner, a "crazy artist" who produces all kinds of pieces, but she is particularly fond of his sculptures. Her sons initially struggled with this new relationship but all that has settled down. "I would never let myself be told what to do in my new relationship. It's my life, after all." Having a new man at her side is really good for her: "Through the separation from my ex-husband I have learned how important it is to pay attention to your own needs and really take them seriously. Nowadays I'm no longer having to fight against my inner voice ..."

"Growing older isn't always fun"

She sometimes finds it difficult to attain the customary serenity that supposedly comes with growing older. Until her early 50s she felt really well from a physical point of view. She went swimming regularly and attended jazz dance classes. "In my mid-50s I noticed that beauty is ephemeral. My connective tissues became weaker, I suddenly didn't feel quite so confident in my swimming costume. I began to feel that in some ways growing older isn't always fun." Cosmetic surgery has not been something she has considered so far: "I haven't had anything done yet, but I wouldn't completely rule out doing something like that. Although I would be so scared of Botox that I definitely wouldn't be the right candidate for that kind of treatment."

And ultimately a woman's self-image is vitally dependent on the kind of environment she moves in: "In certain circles, having work done on your face by your mid-50s is a matter of course and just seems completely normal. But in my circle of friends and acquaintances, there are very few who have had that kind of intervention. And if they have, it was due to something like the annoyance of drooping eyelids rather than to tackle wrinkles."

By contrast she has learned to love her sticking-out ears: "I was teased so often about them as a child I ended up believing that I looked really terrible. Nowadays I've come to terms with them and often I even hook my hair behind my ears to show them off." She also made a conscious decision to embrace her grey hair. On a photo shoot for a hair products company, a young stylist had dyed her hair grey with a pastel pink hue. Barbara says, "It looked great and really fancy – and I didn't even have to do a lot for it." Now she is really happy with her beautiful silver hair in various shades of grey, but she has noticed that she suddenly needs to use rather different make-up: "Grey needs colour. I like to wear lipsticks in various berry shades and I have acquired some striking and colourful reading glasses."

"I haven't got any more relaxed ..."

In other ways too, Barbara hasn't found that old age necessarily makes you any more relaxed or wiser. "More knowledgeable is perhaps a better description," she says. The most important thing for her is to participate actively in life. Particularly to engage with the things that are wrong with our society, such as injustice, racism, and discrimination. Just like in the song "Rise Up", by her favourite musician, Konstantin Wecker. For instance, she finds discrimination against older people "outrageous". Particularly those who live alone and so have little influence. "Often older people are treated as though they are stupid and immature, rather than simply elderly." In these kinds of situations, whether it is at the supermarket or at the doctor's reception desk, she gets stuck right in and confronts inappropriate behaviour. "As long as I can get outraged and get involved, I feel young and alert."

Rise up,
protest,
fight back,
it's never too late!

Rise up,
belong,
love,
and resist!

(From the song
"Rise Up" by Konstantin
Wecker)

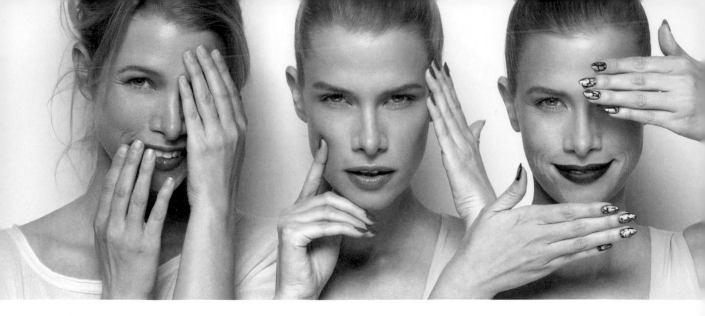

Eye-catching hands

Hands can express feelings, but they also pack a punch. One way or another, they're constantly in use, and without the right care they can easily make us look older. This is how to keep your hands looking good.

Soap opera

Repeated daily hand washing and housework are not good for the delicate skin on your hands, which is naturally poorly endowed with sebaceous glands. The results of excessive exposure to water and cleaning agents are dry, rough, and sometimes reddened hands, with chapped fingertips.

Looking after your hands begins with washing: try to avoid strongly foaming products which usually contain drying sodium laureth sulphate or sodium lauryl sulphate. Instead, select products with gentler surfactants made from sugar or vegetable oil.

A good alternative is an oil-based hand wash, which immediately replaces any lipids that get washed away. When handling household cleaning materials, try to always wear gloves.

Protective measures

To keep hands soft after washing, and also in between, it is vital to use a good hand cream. Look out for ingredients such as vegetable oils and glycerine, urea, aloe vera, and hyaluronic acid, which have intensive moisturizing properties. If your cuticles have a tendency to be dry and to crack, creams and oils designed specifically for nails will soften them again. Pure shea butter also works beautifully. **Tip:** Keep your nail care product on your bedside table and massage a small amount into the skin around your nails every night. Improvement is usually noticeable after just one week.

The finishing touch

Hands that have been well looked after need beautiful nails. For this you either need a professional manicure

Hands are exposed to UV light throughout the year. So always use a hand cream containing sunscreen, and in summer apply a sun cream with SPF 50+ to the backs of your hands.

— or you can achieve it in the comfort of your own home in three steps: push back the cuticle using a little stick with a rubber tip (also known as a cuticle pusher). If the cuticles are tough, first paint on a cuticle remover, and leave to soak in for a minute before removing carefully under warm water with a nail brush. Dry your hands and wait a few minutes. Finally, shape the nails as desired using a high-quality glass, crystal, or ceramic nail file. Whether you prefer your nails rounded or square is a matter of taste, although nails that are filed straight across break more easily than those filed in an oval shape. Remember: don't run the nail file back and forth; always file in a single direction. If you don't want to apply nail varnish, you can use a nail buffer to give the nails a high sheen at the end.

Flecks and grooves

Little blemishes and unevenness sometimes indicate that all is not well in our body. White spots are usually harmless signs of tiny physical impacts on your nails. Longitudinal grooves occur more frequently with age and are also harmless. Transverse grooves, on the other hand, are caused by an overly aggressive approach to nail care and, in rare cases, can be a sign of kidney problems.

If you use a strong colour of nail polish, yellow staining can sometimes occur. Using an undercoat only partly protects against this. In rare cases, such discolouration can be a sign of liver disease. If the nails have a yellowish hue and become woody and brittle, the cause could be a fungal infection, which must be treated with a medicated nail varnish.

Colour for fingers

The crowning glory of a manicure is beautiful nail polish. This is the best way to apply it: shake the bottle well so that the colour pigments are evenly distributed. Wipe off the brush on the neck of the bottle, and swiftly paint the first stripe in the centre of the nail, from the cuticle to the tip of the nail. Then do the same on the right and on the left. Leave this first thin layer of colour to dry for at least five minutes before applying a second or even third coat.

A clear overcoat will give the manicure extra gloss and make it last longer. Any little mistakes can easily be removed by using a corrector pen or a cotton bud dipped in nail varnish remover. Beware that the polish might be superficially dry after about 10 minutes, but it usually only dries fully after half an hour.

PROFESSIONAL HAND REJUVENATION

Wrinkles, pigmentation spots, and visible veins on the backs of our hands sometimes make us look older than we really feel. Nowadays dermatologists have effective treatment methods to make hands look younger. Pigmentation spots can be quickly lasered away without any side effects. Wrinkles and prominent veins on thin skin will be less noticeable after a hyaluronic acid injection, which makes the skin look more youthful and firm (more on this on p.150).

Elegant feet

Feet sometimes have a hard time: cooped up in tights without light or air, mistreated in high-heeled shoes; and still they carry us through the day. Our feet need a bit of tender loving care to make them look elegant again.

Just take a bath

Anyone who spends the whole day on their feet will recognize the problem: by evening our legs and feet feel heavy and sore, our ankles are often swollen. A foot bath provides the ideal relief. Tired feet love invigorating ingredients such as rosemary, mint, camphor, or eucalyptus. For swollen and burning feet, calming herbs such as arnica and camomile will help. If you have a stressful day behind you and want to go straight to bed after your foot bath, three drops of lavender or clary sage essential oil added to the water will guarantee a restorative sleep.

Are your feet prone to sweating? A salt bath can alleviate the condition. Stir 2 tablespoons of sea salt into a litre (1¾ pints) of warm water and then soak your feet for ten minutes.

Remove unwanted dry skin

To keep the soles of your feet soft, they need to be rubbed down every couple of days either with a foot exfoliator or, even better, with a foot file. These usually have two sides: a coarser side for removing the calloused layer of skin and a finer side that is designed to soften the skin. Resist the temptation to use a plane or scalpel on the dead skin: leave these instruments to your chiropodist, or you can literally cut your feet to shreds.

Cutting toenails correctly

In contrast to fingernails, toenails should always be cut or filed straight across to avoid ingrowing toenails. File the edges smoothly and gently round off the corners so they don't catch on your tights.

If you do get an ingrowing nail at some point, as soon as you notice it bathe the foot for five minutes in vinegar (240ml [8fl oz] vinegar to 2 litres [3½ pints] warm water), work on the problem spot with a fine nail file, apply an antiseptic cream or zinc ointment, and protect with a plaster. If the problem has not improved within a couple of days, consult your doctor. A chiropodist can also tackle ingrown nails. He or she will shorten the nail and cover it with a piece of gauze while it heals. Emergency first aid at home: apply a thick layer of dexpanthenol and hydrocortisone (0.5%) ointment, or a blister cream, and cover the nail with a large plaster.

Well nourished

The skin on your feet is drier than on the rest of the body. In addition, the skin can become calloused or rough through the pressure exerted by your bodyweight, from friction and movement, from long periods spent standing or walking, and also from wearing overly narrow shoes. Use a foot cream containing shea butter or glycerine to quickly soften up any dead skin. If the ingredients also include urea (with a concentration of 10%) or salicylic acid, this helps prevent further formation of callouses. If you suffer from dry feet, possibly also with painful cracking on the heels and balls of the feet, you should use a particularly nourishing foot cream containing specialized healing skincare ingredients.

> Relaxing evening ritual: massage your feet ayurvedic-style for two minutes using warm sesame oil. Then put on thin cotton socks – sweet dreams are guaranteed!

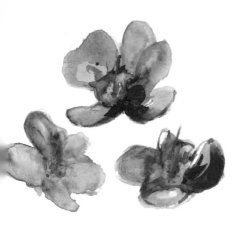

Bunions, blisters, and corns

Overly narrow shoes can cause unattractive and painful pressure points known as corns. These can be removed by a chiropodist in what is normally a painless minor procedure. Alternatively, corn plasters or treatments containing salicylic acid can be used to tackle the problem. Since these latter treatments are highly aggressive, it is important that they do not come into contact with the surrounding skin.

Blisters and areas that have been rubbed sore can be treated with blister plasters, which have a gel layer to keep the affected area damp and so accelerate the healing process. These plasters can also be used as a preventative measure. Remember, our feet get wider as we grow older. Even if you have always worn a size 5½, it's worth trying out a possibly more comfortable size 6 some time.

Similarly, as time goes by, it is common for the big toe to bend towards the other toes. This slanting of the toe causes the ball joint on the inner side of the foot to protrude, which doctors refer to as a hallux valgus (or bunion). An operation is only necessary if there is severe pain. Modern procedures avoid the need for plaster casts, or having to use a walking aid. The patient is able to support gentle pressure on the foot immediately after the operation, and after 4 to 6 weeks normal shoes can be worn again.

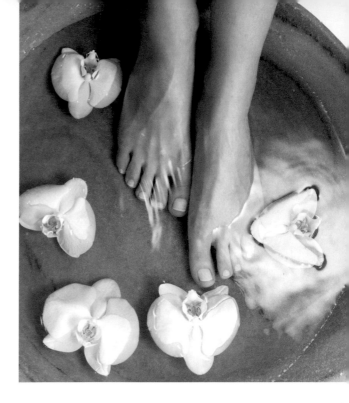

FOOT GYMNASTICS

Your feet have to work pretty hard in high-heeled shoes. These exercises will help compensate.

Roll: Stand barefoot in the door frame. Hold on tight and rise up onto your tiptoes. Hold the position briefly and then roll down onto the whole foot again. Repeat ten times.

Twist: Grasp the front of your foot with one hand and the heel with the other. Twist the front of the foot and the heel gently in opposite directions, as if you were wringing out a towel. Ten repetitions.

Grip: Lay a heavy book onto a thin cloth. Stand a sufficient distance away so that you can just grip one tip of the fabric with your foot. Pull the cloth towards you using your toes. Then switch sides.

Eat to be beautiful

Creams, serums, and cosmetics: there's a lot we can do externally for beautiful skin. But a good diet helps reduce wrinkles and ensure a radiant complexion and good skin tone. Here are the top ten beauty foods.

1 Berries

Blueberries, blackberries, blackcurrants, and raspberries owe their sublime colouring to what are called anthocyanins. In plants these flavonoids are partially responsible for protection from UV light and are effective at catching free radicals. When you eat berries, the body absorbs these cell-protecting substances. According to the latest studies, anthocyanins are significantly more effective as free radical adversaries than the better known vitamins E and C.

2 Pineapple

This tropical fruit is rich in the enzyme bromelain. Enzymes are like little engines that control all kinds of processes in the body, from the immune system to fat metabolism. Bromelain helps break down protein molecules in our food, so they can be used by the body for fat burning. In addition, enzymes help deal with cell waste from old proteins and cholesterol in connective tissues, which can build up and contribute to wrinkles or cellulite.

3 Soya

Soya is the classic super food for golden girls. It contains the substance genistein, which is similar to oestrogen and can gently restore the equilibrium if there are any hormonal imbalances. Soya products also contain vitamin B2, which is good for dry skin. Equally valuable are its unsaturated fatty acids, which help to reduce the risk of cardiovascular disease.

4 Sea fish

Especially oily fish such as tuna, salmon, mackerel, or sardines, which deliver precious omega 3 fatty acids. The body uses these to produce eicosanoids, tissue hormones that help prevent deposits from building up in the blood vessels and so lower the risk of heart attack. This is the number one cause of death among menopausal women, a fact that all too often goes unrecognized. Omega 3 fatty acids also provide protection against chronic inflammatory illnesses such as asthma or arthritis, and even against dementia.

5 Tomatoes

Ripe tomatoes contain high quantities of the red pigment lycopene. This catches free radicals and thus combats premature skin ageing due to UV damage. Tinned tomatoes and tomato purée both contain particularly high concentrations of this protective substance. A bit of fat will help the body absorb it.

6 Olive oil

Olive oil contains many unsaturated fatty acids that help keep blood vessels clear and protect the heart. Healthy fats are also contained in linseed, rapeseed, and avocado oils, as well as in nuts and seeds. Even butter has been rehabilitated lately thanks to its omega 3 fatty acids. Make sure you always get butter from exclusively grass-fed cows, however, as their milk contains around twice the amount of omega 3 fatty acids as milk produced by other cows.

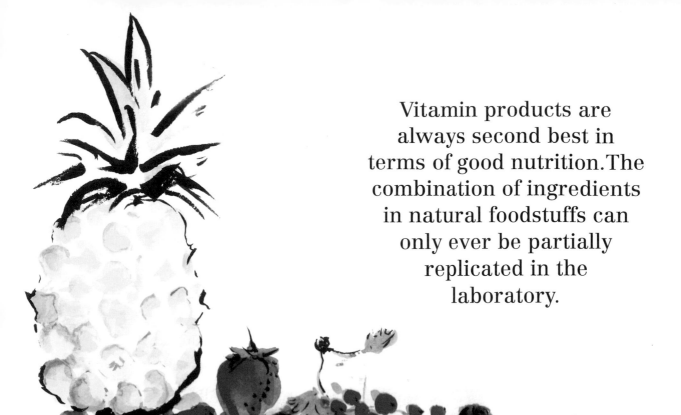

Vitamin products are always second best in terms of good nutrition. The combination of ingredients in natural foodstuffs can only ever be partially replicated in the laboratory.

7 Avocados

Don't worry about the fat content: avocados contain valuable B vitamins and particularly high concentrations of biotin (vitamin B7). These support the body's production of keratin for strong and healthy hair and nails. Pantothenic acid (vitamin B5) is said to lower cholesterol levels and help metabolize fat.

8 Broccoli

This healthy member of the brassica family contains a whole range of ingredients that are important for beauty: secondary plant materials, for instance, which protect cells against free radicals, but also B vitamins to even out fluctuations in mood, calcium to prevent osteoporosis, and vitamin C, which is used in the production of connective tissue.

9 Whole grain products

If you constantly consume products made from white flour, such as white bread, biscuits, and cakes, it is hardly surprising that you are always hungry. Short-chain carbohydrates cause insulin levels to spike dramatically before plummeting again just as quickly – and that results in cravings for more food. In contrast, whole grain products instigate a much slower and less dramatic rise in insulin levels and this makes you feel full for longer.

10 Dried fruit

Dried fruits have a particularly high ORAC value. ORAC stands for Oxygen Radical Absorption Capacity and is a unit of measure for how much protection a foodstuff gives against free radicals and thus also against premature ageing. Frontrunners among the dried fruits are prunes and dried aronia berries (chokeberries).

An afternoon at your home spa

You don't necessarily need an expensive wellness weekend – your own bathroom can be transformed into a feel-good oasis. Here are some top tips for an extended pampering session at home.

Take it slowly

Straight from work, into the bathtub, eyes closed, and now relax please – that just sounds like even more stress. So take your time getting into a relaxed frame of mind. Once home, the first thing to do is to get out of your work clothes. Wrap yourself in a cuddly dressing gown and calmly make yourself a cup of tea. Lavender tea is particularly relaxing, or a fresh lemon verbena tea is also a great start to a pampering session. Switch your mobile onto silent, dim the lighting in the bathroom, and light a few candles or an aroma burner. Essential oils will enhance your inner peace and relaxation, because our mood can be influenced via the limbic system in the brain. For example, citrus oils such as neroli, orange, grapefruit, or lemon have an uplifting effect on your mood, while camomile and lavender are soothing, and rose oil is thought to help stabilize the hormones.

Warm up properly

No one can relax if they are cold. Make sure your home is warm, especially the bathroom. Leave the door closed while you run the bath: that way the room will soon be turned into a warm and humid beauty oasis. Put your towels on a radiator – body oils and lotions should be warmed up in a similar manner. Of course, there is also nothing quite like slipping on a pair of pre-warmed slippers after a pampering session.

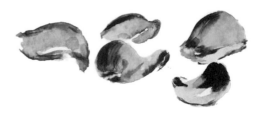

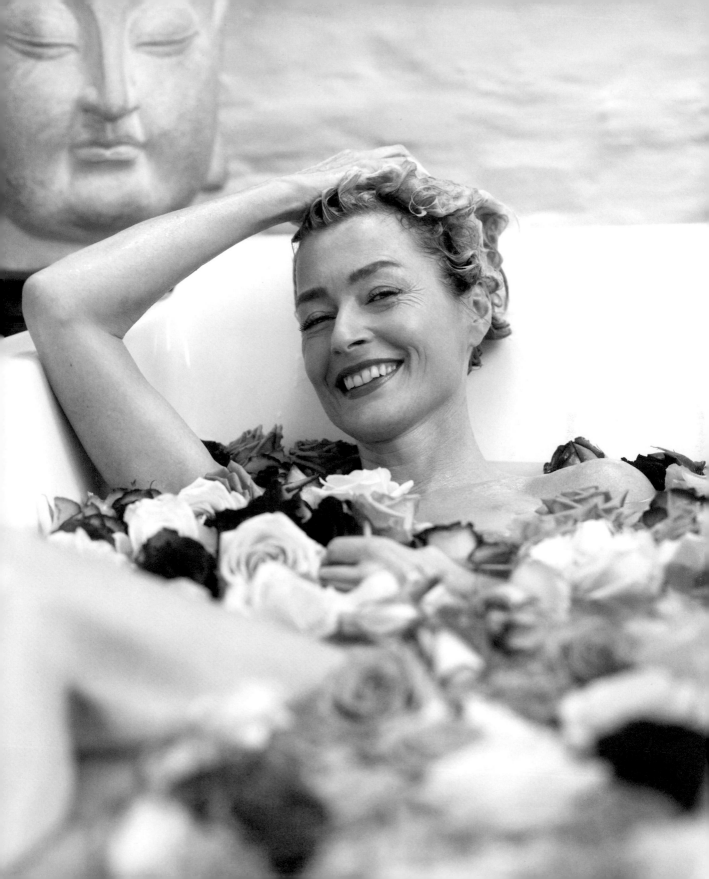

Deep cleanse the pores

Make the most of the time while the bath water is running by giving your complexion a detox treatment. This is especially quick and easy to do using a facial steam bath. Boil some water and pour it into a large bowl or wash basin. Depending on your skin type, you might like to add fragrant fresh or dried herbs or some essential oils. Tea tree oil, lavender, and thyme are ideal if your skin is prone to the occasional blemish; camomile and rose are soothing and moisturizing; and mint has a refreshing impact. After the heat becomes comfortable, you can intensify the effect by placing a towel over your head. (Note: do not use steam baths if you have a tendency towards couperose or rosacea, as it will exacerbate any symptoms.) After the steam bath the pores will be more open, so take advantage and do some eyebrow plucking. The process will be far less painful at this point.

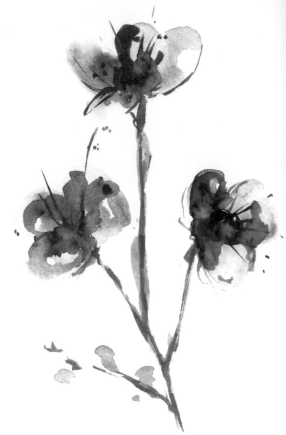

Treats for skin and hair

After the steam bath and before bathing, indulge your skin and hair with a face mask and body scrub. These three beauty concoctions can be made quickly and cheaply at home from ingredients you may well already have in your fridge.

Chocolate face mask
35g (1¼oz) cocoa powder
3 tbsp cream
2 tsp cottage cheese
3 tsp oatmeal
85g (3oz) honey
Stir the ingredients together, apply to face and throat, and leave to work for the duration of the bath. Rinse off with lukewarm water.

Apple pie body scrub
2 tbsp soft brown sugar
2 tbsp white granulated sugar
1 tbsp apple purée
1 pinch ground cinnamon
Stir the ingredients together and use your hand or a flannel to apply the mixture over the whole body using circular movements. If you also want to use the mix on your face, omit the white granulated sugar, as this is too coarse for facial skin. The brown sugar is finer and also readily dissolves in the remaining mask ingredients.

Avocado conditioner
1 avocado, peeled and chopped
2 tbsp cream
1 tbsp honey
Blitz the ingredients using a hand blender and apply to the hair. Put on a disposable shower cap and wrap a warmed towel around your head. Leave to work during the bath, along with the face mask, then rinse out thoroughly with lukewarm water.

Bathed in joy

There are any number of ready-made bath products available. For dry skin, oil baths are best; normal skin will be fine with bubble bath. Effervescent bath bombs briefly transform your bathtub into a sparkling whirlpool. Even better (and far cheaper) are homemade bath products, which have the added bonus that you know exactly what they contain. Here are three options for different occasions:

Warming spice bath

8 tbsp baking powder
2 tbsp sugar
1 tsp ground cinnamon
½ tsp ground ginger
½ tsp ground cloves
Mix the ingredients together and add 2 tbsp of the mixture to warm bath water. Keep the rest of the mixture in a well-sealed glass jar and store in a cool place. The ideal bath temperature is around 39 °C (102°F) ; recommended bathing time is 15 to 20 minutes.

Invigorating orange and rosemary bath

250g (9oz) powdered milk
1 tbsp dried orange peel
1 tbsp dried rosemary
15 drops bergamot essential oil
Mix the powdered milk, orange zest, rosemary, and bergamot oil. Add 8 tbsp of the mixture to the bath water. Ten minutes soaking at a temperature of 36 °C (96.8°F) will be sufficient for an invigorating bath.

Relaxing sea salt bath

1kg (2¼lb) Dead Sea salt
10 drops lavender essential oil
Add the salt to the bathtub and dissolve in very hot water. Then gradually add cooler water until the temperature is between 37 and 38 °C (98.6 and 100.4°F). Only add the lavender oil right at the end. After bathing, shower off briefly in lukewarm water and moisturize the body thoroughly.

And breathe!

After bathing, you can further enhance your spiritual peace and physical relaxation with a simple ayurvedic breathing exercise (pranayama). Close the right nostril using your right thumb. Breath in for 4 seconds through the left nostril. Then close the left nostril too using two fingers on the same hand, and hold your breath for 4 seconds. Now open the right nostril and breathe out for 8 seconds. Breathe in through the right nostril, close both nostrils, hold your breath, and then breathe out through the left nostril. Repeat the exercise beginning with breathing in through the left nostril.

Now there really is just one more thing to do: off you go to the sofa!

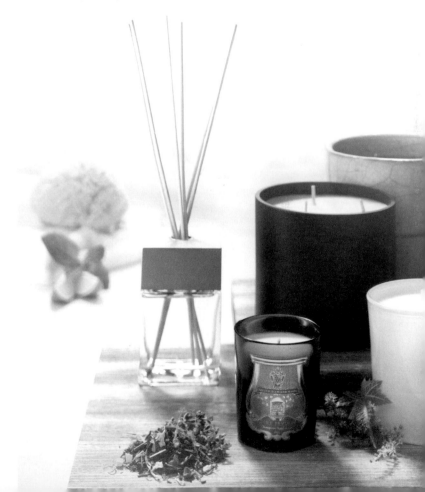

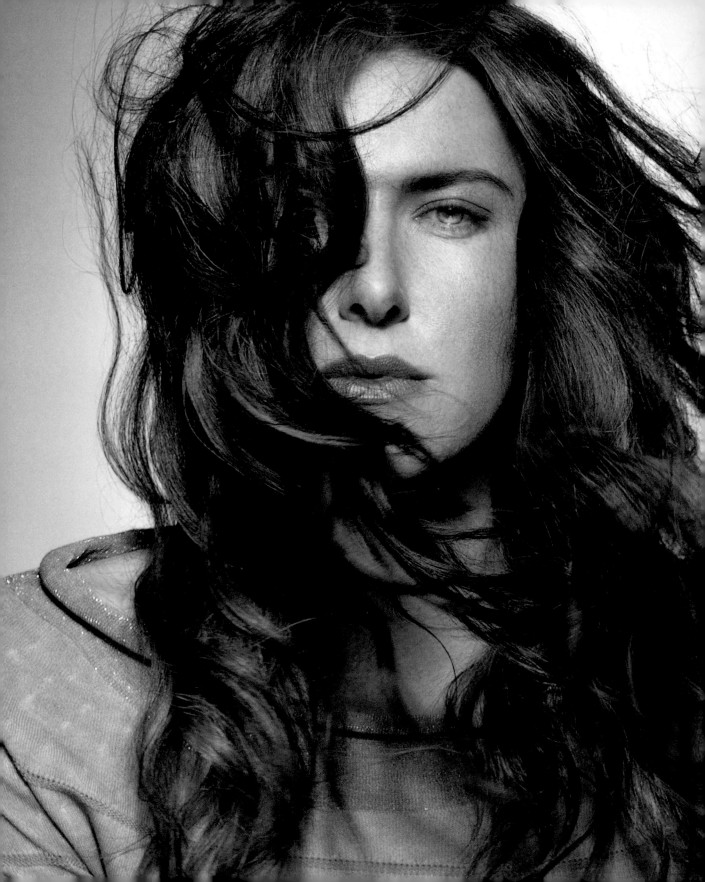

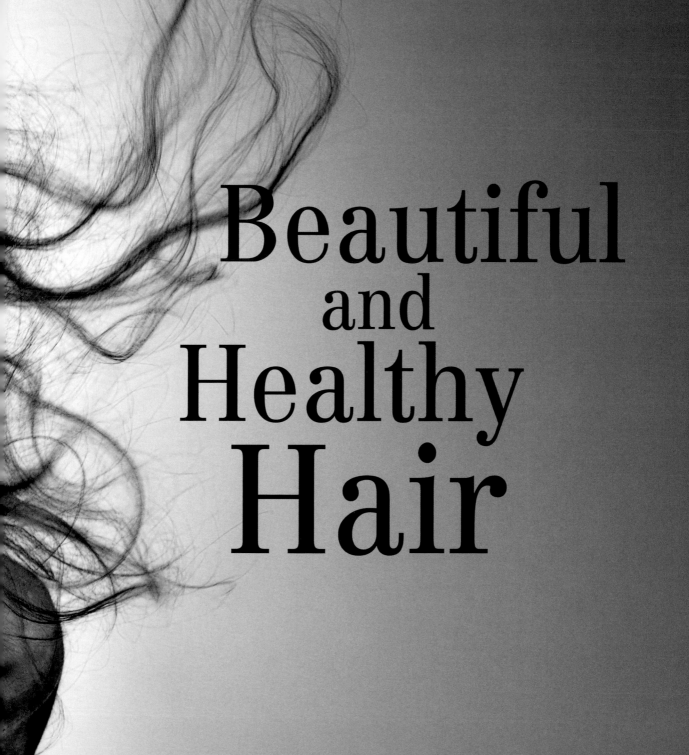

Beautiful
and
Healthy
Hair

Condition & shine for your hair

Not even your hair can escape the ageing process. It becomes thinner and more sensitive, sometimes also losing its shine and volume. But the right conditioning and styling products will ensure it looks thick and gorgeous again.

A matter of cleanliness

A good shampoo forms the basis of your hair care. It should be chosen depending on your type of hair, along with the needs of your scalp. And both of these can vary due to hormonal fluctuations, climate conditions, and with the changing seasons.

Dyed hair requires ingredients to protect the colour from fading and to nourish hair that has been damaged by the colouring process. Dry or brittle hair will benefit from vegetable and silicone oils that coat the hair, restoring its shine. For thinning hair, keratin and other proteins can help make less appear more. Volume shampoos usually gently roughen the hair structure. This makes each individual strand of hair lie slightly further apart from its neighbours, giving an impression of greater body. And grey-silver hair can be given a beautifully rich shade – without any yellow tones – by using a special shampoo that contains violet or blue pigments.

When washing hair, the golden rule is that less is more. Froth up a small amount of shampoo in your hand, briefly massage through the hair, and then thoroughly rinse out using lukewarm water. Any residue can make the hair heavy and lustreless. There is no need to shampoo right down to the ends – these will be washed when you rinse.

> Blow dry your hair sparingly, that means not too hot and with a distance of at least 15cm (6in) between hairdryer and scalp. This prevents dry and brittle hair.

Targeted structural work

With the exception of very short styles, pretty much all hair needs conditioning after washing. The surfactants in shampoo don't just remove dirt particles, they also strip the hair and scalp of some of its protective sebaceous coating. Just as with your shampoo, your conditioner should be chosen based on your hair type.

Conditioner works best if it is applied to towel-dried rather than wet hair. Gently squeeze out your hair after shampooing, ideally with a towel. Leave the conditioner to work for between one and three minutes, as recommended on the packaging. Unlike with other treatments or hair masks, leaving it in for longer brings no additional benefits, because conditioner is formulated to work quickly. Only apply conditioner where the hair actually needs it, namely along the lengths of the hair down to the ends. Conditioner has no place at the roots.

A rule of thumb when rinsing is to rinse for as long as the conditioner was left in to work. Give a final rinse with cold water, because this closes up the hair's cuticle layer, providing extra shine. Ultra-light leave-in conditioners are also available, which are sprayed into the hair after washing. These do not need to be rinsed out and are formulated to avoid making the hair too heavy.

Intensive conditioning

At times your hair needs some special attention. Maybe you've used too many harsh chemical products, or it has just been a bit neglected, or the summer holidays have taken their toll. Hair masks, deep conditioning treatments, and oils have a much more intense impact than everyday conditioner, because they're so highly concentrated. These specialized conditioning treatments can be applied all over the hair. Masks and treatments are then rinsed out thoroughly after the recommended application time. The newer hair oils, on the other hand, are left in and are a great alternative, particularly for unruly or fine hair. They contain a mix of plant oils and "dry" silicone oils, and when dispensed sparingly, they ensure the hair looks silky and elegant without becoming greasy.

Deep conditioning treatments and hair masks are particularly effective in conjunction with warmth: after applying the product, briefly use a hair dryer on the

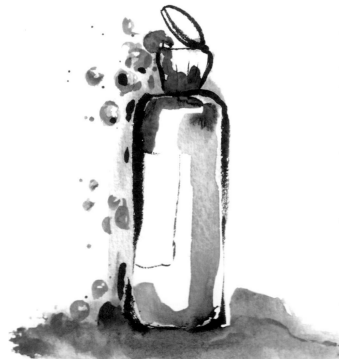

NEED A LITTLE BIT MORE?

During the menopause it is not unusual for hormonal changes to cause hair loss, making the hair look thinner and more sparse. Falling oestrogen levels cause the hair to go into the so-called dormant phase more rapidly than usual, and this results in hair falling out prematurely.

If hormones are the cause of hair loss, your GP may be able to help with treatments containing oestrogen to apply to the scalp, or by prescribing the hormone progesterone. A blood test is used to detect whether there are any additional mineral deficiencies. Final resort: a hair transplant using hairs from the back of the head, which are resistant to hormonal changes.

hair, put on a disposable shower cap (cling film works fine too), and wrap around a towel or hair turban.

The perfect finish

Styling products are very helpful if your hairdo lacks volume and body. There are also certain hairstyles where having more structure in the hair simply looks better. Volume and styling sprays, blow-dry products, and root boosters work by using resins and special polymers that coat each hair with an extremely thin web, making the hair appear thicker. They are sprayed onto towel-dried hair after washing. Most products are suitable for air-drying as well as blow-dried styles, but some are thermo-active, which means that they only work effectively with the warmth from a hairdryer.

There's now a product on the market called volume powder. This is dusted sparingly just at the roots of the hair and, thanks to the resins it contains, the powder becomes very slightly sticky. When gently massaged in with the fingers, this creates extra volume at the roots.

In full colour

Fabulous hair colour is everything: it flatters the complexion, distracts from wrinkles, and can make you look younger. The range of colours, tints, and highlights on offer is extensive and sometimes confusing.

Softly softly: colour shampoos and conditioners

If your hair dye needs a little colour refreshment or your own hair colour could do with a few subtle highlights, colour shampoos and conditioners are the ideal solution. Depending on the brand, they offer varying degrees of pigmentation intensity and simply involve coating the hair shaft with a light to moderate colour film. There is a slight cumulative effect over the course of multiple washes. Colour conditioners generally have a more intense colouring effect than colour shampoos. They can be washed out again after just a few applications of a normal shampoo. Useful tip: with colour shampoos and conditioners, you can test out whether you suit a red or gold tint without having to permanently dye your hair.

Delicate reflections: tints

Tints do not penetrate into the hair like dyes; instead they coat each individual hair with an incredibly thin colour coating. They work without having to be blended with hydrogen peroxide. This makes them especially gentle and they give the hair a beautiful shine thanks to increased light reflection. Unfortunately you can't make your hair go lighter by tinting, but there are beautiful options to play around with using gold, red, or brown highlights.

Whether you prefer foam, fluids, or creams is a matter of personal taste. The original hair colour

> Most women estimate their natural hair colour to be darker than it really is, which can lead to poor results when dyeing hair at home. Ask your hairdresser for appropriate colours.

determines how intense the final colour will be: the lighter the natural hair colour and the darker the tint shade, the stronger the colouring effect will be. If the hair ends are porous or if the hair is damaged, the colour will be absorbed more strongly than in healthy hair. To combat this, apply a conditioning treatment to the ends of the hair before tinting. Depending on the product, tints tend to wash out in two to four washes.

Really long-lasting: dyes

Hair dyes involve significantly more chemicals. The hair's natural colour pigments are stripped out using hydrogen peroxide, allowing new, artificial dyes to penetrate. This means the new colour is firmly embedded in the hair. Even grey hair can be 100% covered using hair dye. So called semi-permanent hair colours are simply a toned-down version. Most semi-permanent dyes will only cover grey up to about 75%. One benefit is that they gradually fade, leaving you with less obvious regrowth than a fully permanent dye. Note that hair colourant can cause a severe allergic reaction in some people, so it's essential to do a patch test in advance, as described on the packaging. Salons also require a test before your first colour appointment.

Bleaching

With a blonde dye you can make the hair up to eight shades lighter. But the chemical process involved is

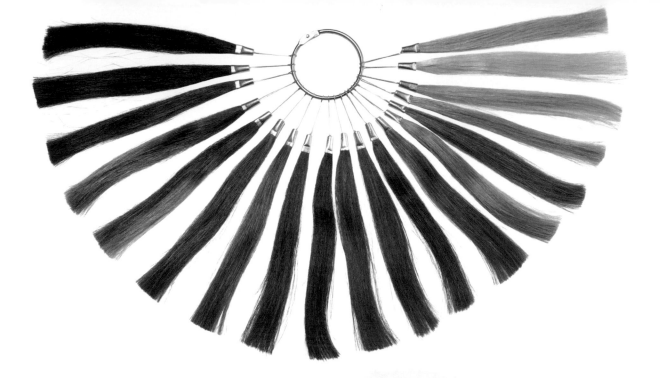

much more damaging to hair than standard dyeing. First the hair's cuticle layer is opened up and a hydrogen peroxide cocktail (which can vary in strength) destroys the natural pigmentation. It is important to adhere to the treatment time recommended on the packaging. If you wash it out too soon, the hair could end up with a red or yellow tone. If the bleach is left to work for too long, on the other hand, the hair can become brittle and porous. Even the best bleaching done by a professional will always damage the hair, so a nourishing conditioning treatment afterwards is essential.

Highlights

Highlights or lowlights can be added to the hair, which can make the hair as a whole look a bit lighter or just add contrast to your natural hair colour. In principle highlights work in the same way as bleaching, but since they are only applied selectively, they are far less damaging to the hair overall. With lowlights, darker or contrasting streaks are introduced by dyeing sections of hair. A combination of darker and lighter streaks can also look wonderful. Be warned: highlights are a time-consuming business that can easily go wrong when attempted at home. To avoid ending up looking like a chipmunk, this is a task best left to your hairdresser.

CORRECT COLOUR CHOICE

For the most natural result possible, you should select a colour no more than two or three shades removed from your natural hair colour. If the jump in colour is too great, your eye colour and eyebrows will expose the deception and the result can easily look unnatural and harsh. With red, copper, and gold shades in particular, you should pay attention to the colour of your complexion. Reddish hues do not look good if your complexion has strong yellow or olive undertones, and they can emphasize any existing red areas on the skin. The ideal candidates for red shades are women with fair skin that is as even as possible and has a delicate pink undertone. Also be careful with darker hair dyes: these can make a fair complexion look even paler. Strong ashy or pearly shades, together with a yellow-toned complexion, can easily look grey, colourless, and old.

From curly to straight

Liberation from the daily battle with curlers, round brushes, or straighteners? What a wonderful thought! Perms and chemical hair straightening make this possible. You can achieve a variety of looks with these treatments.

Less stress for hair

Although the latest perms are far less aggressive than their predecessors and actually condition the hair during the perming process, they cannot function entirely without chemicals. Hair consists of spiral-shaped protein molecules that are connected to each other by means of disulphide bonds. The first step in the perming process involves breaking up a proportion of these disulphide bonds. Then the hair is either shaped into waves by twisting it around curlers, or pulled straight using a hair straightener. A neutralizing solution is applied, which fixes the shape in place for up to four months.

Most treatments today are free from ammonia and only take between 1 and 2 hours. To make sure the process is as kind to the hair as possible, there are special advance conditioning treatments that produce a protective film using keratin and collagen. The perm solution itself also contains nourishing ingredients, such as silk proteins, aloe vera, jojoba oil, the coenzyme Q10, coconut extract, or amino acids to protect the hair's vitality and elasticity. The very latest perm treatments use positively charged particles that lock onto the negatively charged hair, aiming to make it smoother and shinier from within.

You should only ever get a perm done by a professional hairdresser. Home perms without the requisite background knowledge can lead to unsightly

> If you suffer from significant hair loss (more than a hundred hairs per day), you should try to avoid chemical treatments, as these can exacerbate the hair loss.

kinks at the roots, or sections of the hair tips which are not completely wavy. What's more, these kinds of home treatments can be more damaging to the hair than those performed at a salon.

From Afro to full bodied: anything goes

Do you dream of little curls or relaxed waves? This is just as easy to achieve nowadays as adding body or volume at the roots. Even stubborn whorls in the hair can be temporarily tamed. However, hair that is longer than 30cm (12in) is hard to reshape, because it is simply too heavy.

The larger the roller, the weaker the wave. As well as classic perm rollers, there are spiral rollers for corkscrew locks, and conical rollers for particularly natural-looking soft waves. Specialized techniques can add volume to the hair. While a classic perm involves twisting between 80 to 120 thin rollers into the hair, more recent variations involve the hairdresser working with just ten fat curlers up to 7cm (2¾in) in diameter, reshaping the hair in sections. This produces soft waves that you can leave to air dry for a relaxed beach look, wind around rollers for more buoyant curls, or blow-dry completely smooth over a round brush.

Smooth hair that lasts for months

Completely smooth, non-frizzy hair without daily help from straighteners or a round brush? This can be achieved with keratin treatments, also known as a

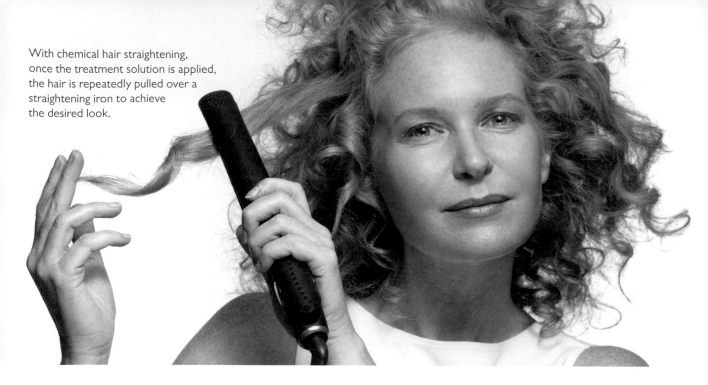

With chemical hair straightening, once the treatment solution is applied, the hair is repeatedly pulled over a straightening iron to achieve the desired look.

Brazilian blow dry or smoothing therapy. These smooth the hair for three to six months, repair it, add shine, and make daily styling much easier.

Just like with perming treatments, none of this is possible without chemicals, because keratin needs a helper to channel it temporarily into the hair. In the past the most common ingredient has been formaldehyde, and its potentially dangerous fumes have led to global controversy over the process. More recent straightening solutions contain different aldehydes or alternative, safer ingredients. It's worth checking with your salon about their process.

How it works: after washing the hair thoroughly, the solution is applied all over, and then the hair is straightened strand by strand using hair straighteners. What might work wonderfully on soft curls, excessive frizz, or unruly hair, is not enough to tame natural really corkscrew hair with stubborn curls. This type of hair needs a straightening treatment that works like a reverse perm and straightens out the strands using active ingredients such as thioglycolic acid or cysteine in conjunction with heat. But be careful: if carried out too frequently, this type of treatment can seriously damage the hair's structure.

AFTERCARE

After a perming or straightening treatment, you should use shampoos and conditioners for damaged or curly hair. The plant oils, silicone, and liquid hair-building blocks these contain will coat the hair in a protective layer and so prevent it becoming brittle, rubbery, and dull.

Leave-in hair masks are also highly practical, as they do not have to be rinsed out again. Once a week you should treat your hair to a nourishing hair mask. This must be left to work for at least half an hour, but you can happily leave it in overnight.

Tip: Avoid getting your hair dyed for at least 4 weeks after having a perm or straightening treatment, as this imposes a double burden on the hair. Non-chemical tints or colour shampoos are fine.

Did you know ...?

These are the questions women ask me most often – and my tips!

1 **Is there any way of hiding puffiness under the eyes?**
Unfortunately this cannot be completely masked by make-up, but you can use concealer to even out the complexion so that any puffiness is less noticeable and appears to blend into the background (see p.17). If you only get occasional puffiness in this area, it's probably caused by water retention. In this case, it helps to consume as little salt and alcohol in the evening as possible, and to sleep with your head on an elevated pillow. Also helpful is professional facial lymphatic drainage.

2 **My foundation settles into my wrinkles – what can I do to stop this?**
Use a liquid, highly pigmented product, and apply it in as thin a layer as possible. Foundation can be applied lightly using a sponge, which reduces the risk of it settling into any small creases.

3 **What is the best way to disguise pigmentation spots, red, or bluish veins?**
The magic word here is layering. This involves applying a thin, liquid foundation in multiple layers as thinly as possible onto skin that has been well moisturized beforehand. Where there are significant blemishes, apply an additional layer.

4 **My eyebrows don't grow properly any more – what can I do to make them fuller?**
It is relatively straightforward to make the eyebrows appear thicker by using an eyebrow powder or by dotting them with an eyebrow pencil (see pp.44–45). If the eyebrows are really thin due to excessive plucking or through illness, there is the option of having an eyebrow transplant. This involves taking hairs, including the follicle, from the rear of the head and implanting them in the eyebrow area. The good news: once an eyebrow transplant has been performed, the hair will never fall out again. But the shape of the brows cannot be altered afterwards and the hair will need trimming once a week as it grows more vigorously than natural eyebrows. This procedure is also pretty expensive.

5 **Sea green or violet – only young women can wear those, right?**
The principle is: soft colours – soft effects, strong colours – strong effects. Sadly, many women are fearful of strong colours once they reach their mid-40s. But accentuating with a strong colour, e.g. on the lips or finger nails, can give depth and contour, and thus also radiance and freshness.

6 **How do you make droopy eyelids less noticeable?**
With the correct make-up techniques, droopy eyelids can be made to look seductive and sexy. Here are the tricks and tips for a fantastic look:

• When applying foundation, don't forget the eyelid. The lid should be free of any grease, then the eye shadow will adhere better.

• Fill in the eyebrows very subtly with a relatively pale eyebrow powder. Harsh lines will only emphasize any droopiness.

• Don't use too pale a colour on the main part of the eyelid, as this further emphasizes the droopy lid. Instead, go for a medium shade as a highlight.

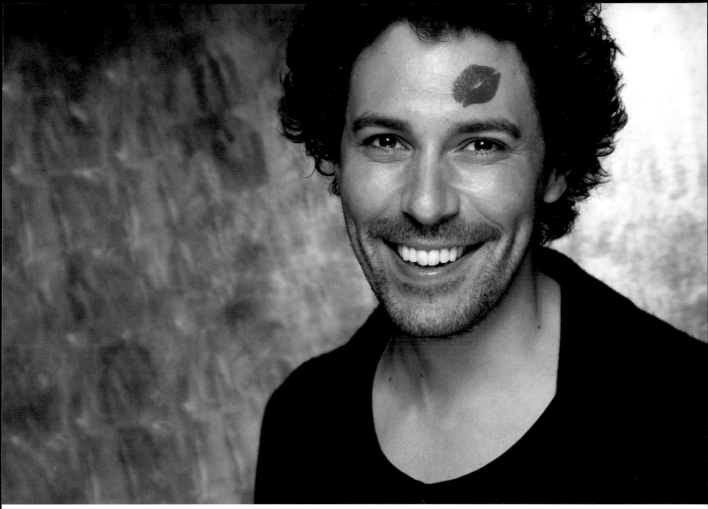

Cool colours go well with lavender tones; for warm colours and blue eyes, I recommend a bronze shade.

- Now look straight ahead in the mirror and add eye shadow in a darker tone, for example a dark brown, to the area precisely above the centre of the eyelid highlight.

- Then use your ring finger to carefully lift the overlapping lid upwards from the eyebrow until the eyelid crease is visible, and shade this in with a dark eye shadow. To do this, use an angled eye shadow brush and then soften the effect with an eye shadow blender, so that there are no harsh edges. Take care not to shade too strongly towards the eyebrows, as this looks too heavy above the eye.

- A finely drawn kohl line right up against the upper eyelash line makes the eyelashes appear thicker.

- To enlarge the eyes even further, dab some highlighter directly under the eyebrows to lift them and let the eyes shine.

- Finally, curl the eyelashes with an eyelash curler (important!) and add plenty of mascara.

Try applying this make-up step by step to just one eye first to really see the difference. You'll be astounded at the effect!

7

I always use lipsticks in subtle shades of pink. Could I also wear red lipstick?
Absolutely! Any woman can wear red lipstick. Just follow these ground rules:

- Only emphasize one part of your face – either eyes or lips. That looks more interesting and classy than trying to draw attention to both.

- Gently rub the lips down with a damp flannel to remove any flakes of dead skin. This will give you an even end result.

- Always moisturize dry lips beforehand.

- Outline the lips using a colourless lip liner.

- It is crucial to apply red lipstick with a brush. Only perfectly shaped red lips look beautiful and stylish.

- It all comes down to the correct shade of red, which should be chosen to match your skin tone. Cool colour types – who have a rosy pink tone to the skin – suit red shades that have a hint of blue. Anyone with a yellow-toned or olive complexion is better off using yellow- or orange-based reds. Be warned, though, that these can make the teeth look yellow.

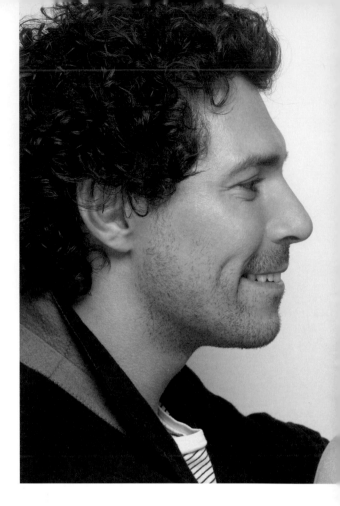

8

I don't have many eyelashes and they are very thin. What can I do?
Volume mascaras are the simplest solution. Make sure you select a product where the applicator separates the individual lashes well, otherwise you'll get a clumping effect that will make your eyelashes look even more sparse than before you started. Other solutions include eyelash extensions, and thickening with individual lashes, or eyelash serums that boost growth, making the lashes longer, thicker, and darker in around 4 weeks.

9

I have little wrinkles around my mouth and very thin lips. What is the best way of using make-up to subtly make them look bigger?
Please never apply colour over the contours – that kind of trickery is guaranteed to go wrong and the result can look truly grotesque! It is better to give your lips a bit of a boost as follows:

- If you are using foundation, include the lips.

- Next apply a bit of powder to the lips.

- Outline the lips using a nude shade of lip liner. Go around the edges of the lips and a tiny bit over.

- Dab a bit of shimmering highlighter on the cupid's bow of the upper lip: this makes the lips look larger and fuller.

- The golden rule is: matte lipsticks make the lips look smaller; bright, glossy lipsticks make them appear bigger. So finish off by filling in your lips with a brilliant iridescent lip gloss.

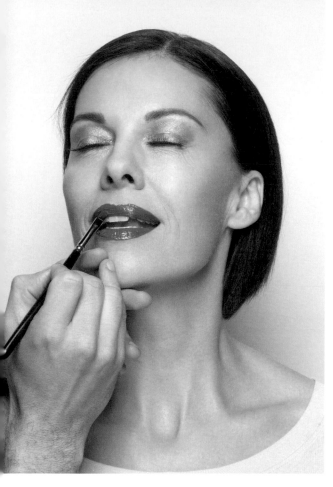

- Use a light-reflecting concealer under the eyes.

- Only use powder in the T-zone of the face; the rest of your skin should retain its natural glow.

11 **Trendy colours – are they for me too?**
You do not have to join in with every trend. Having said that, every season there are various "must haves" and something appropriate for everyone. Trendy colours can be incorporated in so many different ways and can be adapted to suit any style.

12 **Can I still wear eyeliner at my age?**
Eyeliner suits any age. As the area becomes softer and more wrinkled, I would recommend kohl or kajal over a more precise eyeliner (see p.37). Liquid eyeliner can look a little harsh, while kohl is softer, especially when smudged, and imparts a more youthful and dramatically glamorous look. It also looks great if applied directly to the waterline of the lower eyelid, just as they wear it in the East. But I would recommend avoiding black kohl in favour of colours such as taupe, silvery grey, and forest green. These look softer on more mature eyes.

10 **What can I do to combat pale, tired skin?**
In the morning lay a lukewarm flannel as a compress on the skin to open up the pores and stimulate circulation. Remove the flannel and apply a serum to the still slightly damp skin. This helps the serum bond particularly well with the skin, protects against loss of moisture, and forms the perfect base for applying your make-up. An exfoliation treatment is also appropriate for lifting the greyish fog caused by loose flakes of dead skin. When applying foundation, remember:

- Even out varying skin tones and colour differences in stressed skin areas with some light foundation and apply shimmering highlights to the cheekbones, bridge of the nose, and inner corners of the eyes: this gives a particularly beautiful glow.

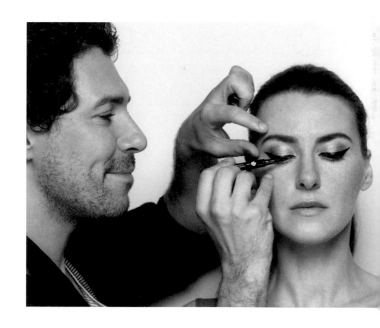

Hello Doc!

When fine lines become deep creases, the next question is: should I have something done? Gentle, almost painless, and minimally invasive treatments are highly fashionable. Get some advice from a specialist.

Acid smoothing: chemical peels

Chemical peels range in intensity from delicate to harsh. They all function in the same way: a chemical reaction causes the removal of several layers of skin. This process strips away any loose, old flakes of skin from the surface and, particularly with the more highly concentrated peeling treatments, stimulates cell renewal in the deeper skin layers. Superficial fruit acid peels in lower concentrations leave the skin looking slightly fresher and healthier. When applied, you just feel a very slight burning sensation. After a specific treatment time the fruit acid is neutralized and then washed off.

Afterwards the skin is briefly slightly red, but you can apply foundation straight away. Moderate to deep fruit acid peels can also smooth out little wrinkles and acne scars and lighten pigmentation spots. These must only be applied by a dermatologist, while superficial fruit acid peels may also be used by beauticians.

After a deep fruit acid peel, the skin will be noticeably reddened for several days and may flake to some extent. Beneath these flakes a new, smoother, healthier skin will appear, but this is initially highly sensitive and must, therefore, be protected from the sun with a sun protection factor of 50+.

Really deep peels using trichloroacetic acid (TCA; used in the case of severe acne scarring or deep creasing) are painful and are applied either under a local anaesthetic or using sedation. Afterwards the skin has a severely red, raw surface that must be protected using ointments and a film dressing.

Moisture combats wrinkles: fillers

In recent years, of all the filler substances used to combat wrinkles, only hyaluronic acid has become established. This substance is already present in our connective tissue and thus is well tolerated by the body. Allergic reactions to it are virtually unheard of.

Hyaluronic acid occurs in different versions, adapted to suit every type of wrinkle. There are especially thin liquid preparations with tiny gel particles, to give the whole face a fresher appearance. Other formulations have larger particles and are designed for targeted application where greater volume is desired, perhaps around the lips or the cheeks. To avoid the hyaluronic acid being broken down too rapidly by the body, it should also be cross-linked.

Injecting wrinkles with hyaluronic acid is virtually painless, often the substance is mixed with a local anaesthetic or the doctor applies an anaesthetic ointment before treatment. After the injection there can be slight swelling or redness at the puncture point, and bruising (haematoma) is also possible. The body breaks down hyaluronic acid within 6 to 12 months, at which point supplementary injections are possible.

Smooth out those lines: botulinum toxin A

Without a doubt, Botox polarizes opinion: there is no other substance to rival it for treating expression lines, such as frown lines on the forehead – and no other substance causes such concern for those using it. Ultimately botulinum toxin A is, exactly as the name suggests, a neurotoxin formed from bacteria. However, in cosmetic medicine it is used in extremely low doses that cannot inflict any great harm on the body.

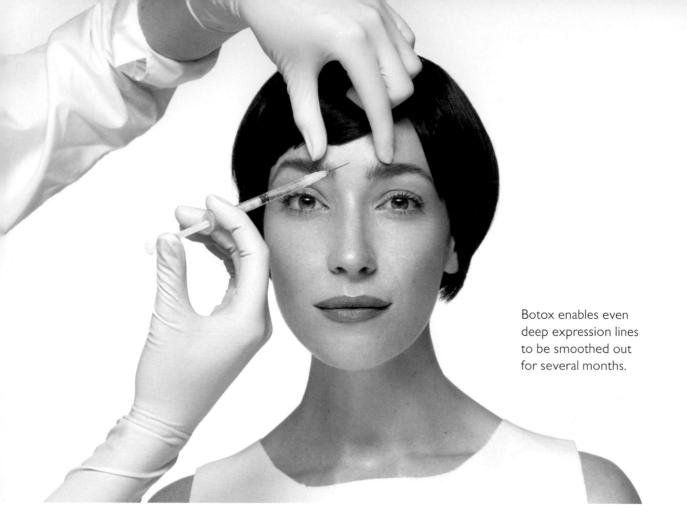

Botox enables even deep expression lines to be smoothed out for several months.

Botox inhibits the release of the neurotransmitter acetylcholine, which issues the command for muscles to constrict. If this message is absent, muscles stay relaxed. In other words, furrowing your brow, for instance, becomes completely impossible for between 4 to 6 months after treatment, and the area remains smooth. Botox is not just used in the forehead area to treat frown lines; it can also be used around the eyes to make them appear more open, and it can combat sagging at the corners of the mouth.

In very rare instances Botox treatment can be associated with some transient facial paralysis, such as droopy eyelids. Sometimes treatment is immediately followed by a short-term headache.

Heat treatments for firmer skin: radio frequency, laser, and ultrasound

For a number of years, so-called "skin tightening" procedures have been gaining currency as an alternative to surgical facelift treatments. While other techniques prioritize reducing wrinkles, these focus on making the skin firmer through the application of heat.

One of the most popular methods involves equipment using a combination of infrared light and radio frequency energy to heat connective tissues to between 40 and 45°C (104 and 113°F) . This warming triggers a mild inflammatory skin reaction, which, in turn, stimulates the fibroblast cells (connective tissue cells) to regenerate collagen. In this way, wrinkles are effectively padded out from within, ensuring a smoother, firmer skin tone. All that is felt during

The new lifting techniques can tone your face without use of a scalpel, virtually pain-free, and without requiring time off work.

treatment is a mild sensation of heat or warmth. Slight redness on the skin directly afterwards is not uncommon, but can be concealed immediately using foundation. The final result, however, doesn't really become apparent until after a period of 3 to 6 months. This is how long it takes for the connective tissue fibres to be completely regenerated.

Power peel with water and air: jet peels and HydraFacials

No glamorous Hollywood star would be without so-called red carpet treatments before special occasions. These kinds of treatments have maximum wow factor and minimum side effects. You can be perfectly presentable straight afterwards, and there is no danger of any longer term redness or other irritation to the facial skin.

In jet peel treatments a special water and gas mix is blasted at top speed onto the skin. It does not hurt at all – in fact it feels pleasantly cooling – and it works a bit like an extremely gentle sandblast exfoliation. Loose, dead flakes of skin are removed, allowing new healthy skin to shine through. Afterwards your complexion will be as radiant as if it had been freshly polished.

A HydraFacial treatment works similarly. But in this procedure a very delicate abrasive attachment physically removes flakes of skin, while power serums, selected to meet the individual's requirements, are transported deep into the skin. Both treatments are also suitable for very sensitive skin with a tendency towards couperose or rosacea.

Needlework toning: needling

This treatment might seem a bit brutal, but it produces excellent results. A roller or pen with extremely fine needles measuring 1.5 mm to 2 mm in length is drawn across the skin, which must have previously had an anaesthetic cream applied. The minuscule punctures to the uppermost skin layer release various growth factors that stimulate regeneration of the connective tissues. This makes the skin firmer, more toned, and smoother.

The treatment is even more effective if accompanied by topical application of a mix of hyaluronic acid, vitamins, and amino acids. Beware though, that after needling the skin is usually very red, and the many tiny punctures sometimes bleed slightly too. The whole thing looks worse than it really is. The skin punctures and bleeding are intentional and heal very rapidly.

Flashlight on pigmentation spots: lasers

A person's true age can be detected from their hands. Unfortunately this observation has an element of truth about it. There is barely another part of the body that is so exposed to UV light and other environmental effects. In addition, as a person ages there is a natural decline in subcutaneous fatty tissues. The hands become bonier and blue veins show through the skin.

Ruby or alexandrite lasers can be used to remove dark spots on the backs of the hands. Usually pigmentation spots disappear after just one session. After treatment the brown spots initially go white, they then change colour over the course of a couple of days (depending on skin type, they may go dark brown or black), and a thin crust will form. After about 2 weeks the crust falls off to reveal skin with even pigmentation. It is important to resist scratching at the lasered skin area during this period, and frequent hand washing can be counterproductive. You should also avoid sunshine and tanning salons and after the initial fortnight the backs of the hands should be protected daily for around 8 weeks using a sunblock with SPF 50+.

Bony hands can be given a bit of padding to make them look younger. This is where hyaluronic acid comes into play. Any sunken areas can be gently injected (having previously applied an anaesthetic to the backs of the hands) and the doctor can stretch them out using their fingers. A second treatment after 4 weeks is recommended.

Coldness combats unwanted padding: cryolipolysis

Making fat cells cold. That is literally what's involved in so-called cryolipolysis. This technique is an ideal choice if the infamous few extra pounds on your stomach or thighs just won't budge, even with exercise or weight loss. The cold treatment won't work for the seriously overweight.

In cryolipolysis the tissue is sucked in using a vacuum and chilled down to 4°C (39°F) for one hour. The cold damages fat cells, resulting in a breakdown of the fatty tissue, while the subcutaneous tissue is simultaneously made firmer.

The procedure is virtually painless: you just feel a strong cold sensation for the first few minutes, and then nothing. Temporary reddening and swelling are possible after treatment. A feeling of numbness may persist for up to 8 weeks. One session is usually sufficient to permanently eliminate these fatty deposits.

LID CORRECTION FOR AN ALERT LOOK

Even around the eyes, gravity eventually wins out. Droopy eyelids often give a forlorn and tired impression. There is a minor procedure that doesn't require hospital admission and is relatively low risk, which can gently open up the eyes and make the whole face look significantly younger. It involves using a scalpel or laser to remove excessive skin from the upper eye lid; the scar will subsequently be concealed within the eyelid crease.

After the procedure, minor bruising and swelling is normal but there is virtually never any discomfort. Like most cosmetic procedures, this is unlikely to be covered by the NHS or private health insurance.

Essential tools

1 Large lip brush
The flat head of the brush enables you to apply colour quickly and evenly in one go.

2 Small lip brush
This finer brush facilitates precise application to create an accurate lip line.

3 Fan eyelash brush
Using a fan-shaped brush, you can apply mascara specifically to the base of the lashes. This defines and separates the lashes.

4 Eyebrow brush
Indispensable: a spiral-shaped nylon brush to shape the eyebrows. You can also use a mascara wand.

5 Eyeliner and eyebrow brush
Its angled shape makes it perfect for precise eyeliner application or for filling in eyebrows.

6 Highlighter brush
Perfect for adding eyeshadow highlights in the inner corner of the eye or below the eyebrows.

7 Eyeshadow brush
Enables comprehensive, even application of eyeshadow. The compact bristles prevent particles from ending up beneath the eyes.

8 Eyeshadow blender
This tool is ideal for blending eyeshadow.

9 Finishing brush
This soft brush enables you to add precise highlights once you have finished applying your make-up.

10 Foundation brush
This is great for the smooth application of liquid foundation and allows you to blend in any shading or highlighting.

11 Powder brush
This brush size is perfect for fixing liquid foundation and giving it a matte appearance.

12 Concealer brush
Cream and liquid concealers can be applied precisely and evenly using this brush.

13 Blusher brush
Thanks to the angled, rounded shape this brush will blend blusher without borders or harsh edges.

14 All-round blender
Too much eyeshadow or foundation, blotchy blusher? This all-rounder will even everything out again.

15 Eyelash curler
Brings a curl to your lashes, giving a more alert expression. It should have rounded edges.

16 Tweezers
High-quality tweezers will have well-polished tips. The bevelled shape enables even the finest hairs to be seized firmly.

17 Make-up sponge
Dry or slightly moistened – this can be used to evenly apply liquid foundation.

18 Cotton buds
For correcting little make-up mistakes.

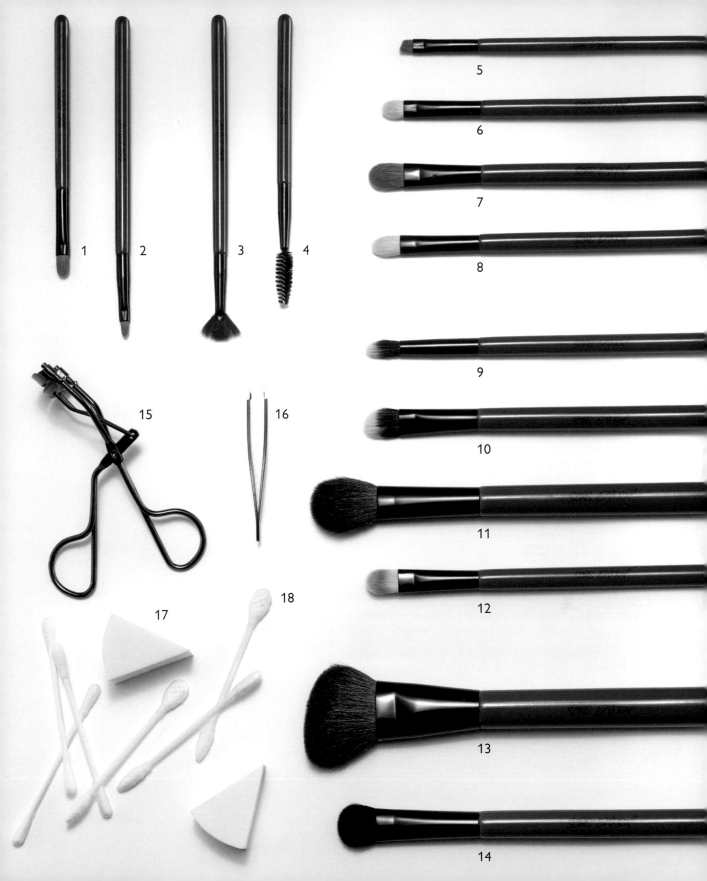

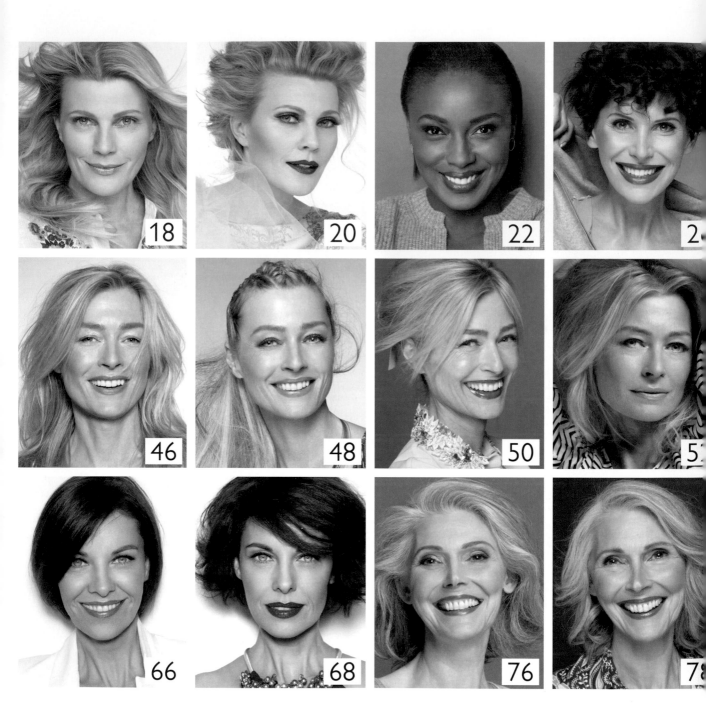

18

20

22

2

46

48

50

5

66

68

76

78

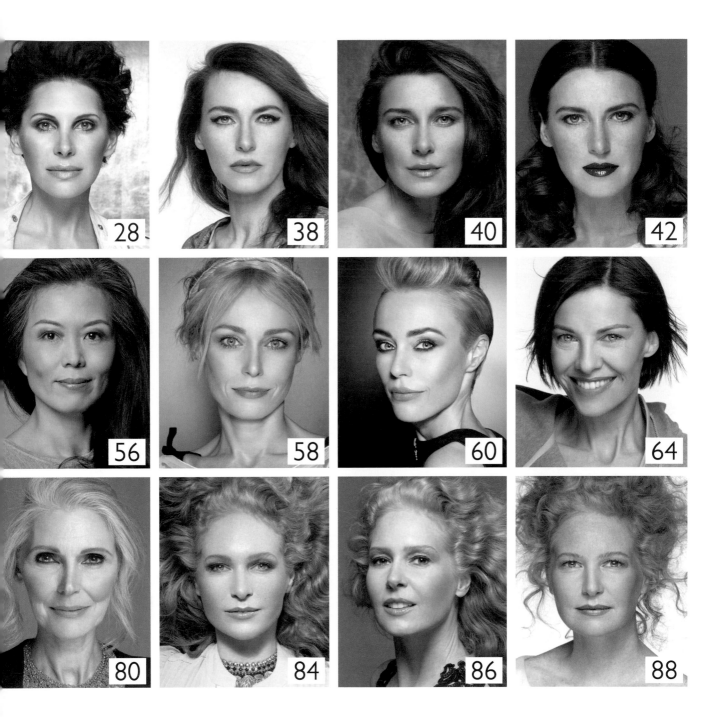

28

38

40

42

56

58

60

64

80

84

86

88

INDEX

ACKNOWLEDGEMENTS

First of all, I would like to thank all the women who have inspired me over the last few years to produce this book. 40+ is a massive and exciting topic.

Almuth, Anna, Barbara, Caprice, Carolina, Esther, Eveline, Ingrid, Julia, Kerry, Marion, Martina, and Marzena – thank you. Each of you in your own way has hugely impressed me and I hope there will be many more mutual projects for us again in future.

A huge thank you is owed to my creative team who supported me so perfectly throughout the entire production process: Denise and Ulf Krentz, who took the sensational photos and have captured on camera my eye for beauty; Natasha Bulstrode and Katja Stawarz, who calmly and patiently assisted me with the hair and make-up; the team assistants Julia Watkins and Lisa Speer, who were an indispensable and inexhaustible source of help for all the make-up artists; Sabine Berlipp, who created the styling to go with the looks I designed. And Silke Amthor, who made my input readable.

I would also like to thank the team from DK publishers Germany: especially Monika Schlitzer for her faith in my idea; Andrea Göppner and Caren Hummel for their perseverance until the blueprint was complete; and all those who were so dedicated in looking after my book behind the scenes.

Emphatic thanks also to the brand creators at BrandFaktor – Sigrid Engelniederhammer and Annette Ballhausen – your commitment and vision are world class. Thank you.

And thank you, of course, to my family!!

Every single person who has helped me produce this book has put their heart and soul into the project – and I am sincerely grateful to all of you.

Thank you to the labels who supported the styling: Fashion ID (Christian Berg Women, Jake*s, Mariposa, Montego, Review, etc.), Adidas, Allude, Almendra Ximello, American Apparel, Balmain, Björn Becker, Bread and Boxers, Cividini, COS, E.M.M.A. Antwerpen, Guido Maria Kretschmer, GY'BELL, H&M, Icon Eyewear Europe, Irene Luft, Jimmy Choo, Joop!, Joyce & Girls, Just Cavalli, Konplott, LAXX Professional Eyelashes, Mango, Marcel Ostertag, Miranda Konstantinidou, Monies, New Yorker, Opus, Paffen Sport, R 95th, Rita Lagune, Sisley, Susanne Bommer, Talbot Runhof, Van Laack, VAVA, Weekday, Zara.

BORIS ENTRUP

Boris Entrup began his career by training as a hair stylist, working internationally as an assistant to renowned and prestigious hair and make-up artists, before setting up independently. Since 2007 Boris Entrup has been the exclusive make-up artist for Maybelline New York. Alongside this expert role, he currently works as an independent make-up artist and beauty expert for numerous international companies, on photo shoots, TV productions, fashion shows, and for magazines – his knowledge and passion are constantly in demand.

His clients include not only models from the fashion and beauty industries, but also prominent celebrities who seek his expertise for their public appearances. The inspiration he provides as a passionate and creative make-up artist helps shape current trends and he translates international catwalk trends for everyday use.

BORIS ENTRUP'S MANAGEMENT TEAM

BRANDFAKTOR – the brand creators
Sigrid Engelniederhammer
Georgenstraße 5
80799 Munich
Tel: +49 89 38 37 71 50
www.brandfaktor.com

DENISE & ULF KRENTZ

The wonderful Denise and Ulf Krentz have been working together as a photography team for almost 20 years. Their very first project together was exhibited at the Ludwig Forum for international art. In subsequent years they have produced numerous photographs for international cosmetics clients and magazines.

Denise Krentz: "The important thing for us with this book was to really capture the spirit of the women. Beauty knows no age. Happy and honest moments have a particular radiance." www.krentzphotography.com

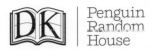

Head of make-up and hair Boris Entrup
Make-up Natasha Bulstrode, Katja Stawarz
Make-up assistants Julia Watkins & Lisa Speer (Famous Face Academy)
Photography Denise Krentz & Ulf Krentz
Digital Operator Tom Reißig
Photography assistant Daniel Rau
Fashion styling Sabine Berlipp, www.blossommanagement.de
Styling assistant & stills Dorothee Krauhausen, www.dk-styling.com
Text Silke Amthor
Editing Julia Niehaus
Illustrations Anna Kuen
Design Gudrun Bürgin

For DK Germany
Publisher Monika Schlitzer
Senior editor Caren Hummel
Project support Andrea Göppner, Caren Hummel
Producer Dorothee Whittaker
Production Christine Rühmer
Production coordinator Arnika Marx

For DK UK
Editor Kate Berens
Translator Alison Tunley
Senior editor Kathryn Meeker
Senior art editor Glenda Fisher
Producer, pre-production Robert Dunn
Producer Stephanie McConnell
Creative technical support Sonia Charbonnier
Managing editor Stephanie Farrow
Managing art editor Christine Keilty

First published in Great Britain in 2017 by
Dorling Kindersley Limited
80 Strand, London, WC2R 0RL

Copyright © 2016 Dorling Kindersley Verlag GmbH
Text copyright © 2016 Boris Entrup
Photography copyright © 2016 Denise & Ulf Krentz
Translation copyright © 2016 Dorling Kindersley Limited
A Penguin Random House Company
10 9 8 7 6 5 4 3 2 1
001–298757–Jun/2017

A CIP catalogue record for this book
is available from the British Library.
ISBN: 978-0-2412-8344-8

Printed and bound in China

All images © Dorling Kindersley Limited
For further information see: www.dkimages.com

A WORLD OF IDEAS:
SEE ALL THERE IS TO KNOW

www.dk.com

MODEL AGENCIES

Brüderchen & Schwesterchen GmbH
Luegallee 7
40545 Düsseldorf
www.bruederchenundschwesterchen.com
Model: Barbara

Favorite Faces
Casting + Model Booking
Schanzenstraße 31 – Schanzenhaus
51063 Cologne
www.favorite-faces.de
Models: Almuth, Ingrid

Mega Model Agency
Brodersweg 3
20148 Hamburg
www.megamodelagency.com
Model: Eveline

Model Pool International Model-Management
GmbH
Elisabethstr. 14
40217 Düsseldorf
www.model-pool.de
Models: Marion, Marzena

NOTOYS Modelagency GmbH
Schwanenmarkt 12
40213 Düsseldorf
www.notoys.de
Models: Esther, Kerstin, Martina

ZAV-Künstlervermittlung Köln
Innere Kanalstr. 69
50823 Cologne
zav.arbeitsagentur.de
Models: Carolina, Julia

Boris Entrup **brushes and products** are available
at: www.be-products-company.com